W9-BUW-640

IN SELF-DEFENSE

IN SELF-DEFENSE

Steven B. Mizel

Peter Jaret

HARCOURT BRACE JOVANOVICH, PUBLISHERS

SAN DIEGO NEW YORK LONDON

Grateful acknowledgment is given to Random House, Inc. for permission to reprint an excerpt from *A Place to Come to* by Robert Penn Warren. Copyright © 1977 by Robert Penn Warren.

Library of Congress Cataloging in Publication Data

Mizel, Steven B.
In self-defense.

Bibliography: p.
Includes index.
1. Immune response. 2. Immunity. I. Jaret, Peter.
II. Title.
QR186.M59 1985 612.7'9 84-12906
ISBN 0-15-144552-4

Designed by G.B.D. Smith
Printed in the United States of America
First edition
A B C D E

To Billie Mizel, and to Ellen and Ralph Jaret

It was our good fortune to have Susan Jaret McKinstry's comments on many of these chapters. Steven Peterson's insightful comments and suggestions are reflected on virtually every page. We would like to thank them both.

S.B.M. and P.E.J.

CONTENTS

IN SELF-DEFENSE

o n e

THE BODY UNDER SIEGE

To be or not to be, that is the question.

WILLIAM SHAKESPEARE

At every moment of its existence, the human body is locked in a life and death struggle for survival. The enemies are silent, unseen, and everywhere around us—viruses too small to be detected by the most powerful light microscopes, bacteria capable of damaging the lining of the lungs or destroying the tissues of the heart, single-celled protozoa and other microscopic organisms that carry within them the capacity to disable or destroy us. Several hundred viruses are known to infect the human body. Hundreds more potentially destructive bacteria swarm in the world around us—borne on the air or carried in the water, teeming in the soil, transmitted through contact with other living things. Indeed, most of us already carry within our bodies organisms which, if unchallenged, would destroy us.

In the face of such a threat, it is a wonder that we survive at all. And the wonder is the human immune system.

Our fight against disease has been fought on many fronts, for many thousands of years. But only within the past decade have we begun to understand the complex and powerful strategies by which the body defends itself against infection and disease. Revolutionary advances in the science of immunology have helped researchers trace the picture of an intricate system of surveillance and defense, operating on the most basic level of cell against cell, by which the body detects and destroys disease-producing organisms. We have identified vast armies of specialized blood cells constantly circulating throughout the tissues of the human body and capable of recognizing and destroying any one of hundreds of thousands of potential enemies. We have even begun to decipher the way these cells communicate—the chemical language they use to signal each other, alert nearby cells, and set in motion the complex defense mechanisms that will destroy the invader.

At work, the system is one of the sustaining marvels of life.

Consider the hepatitis B virus, nothing more than a simple circular strand of DNA—inert genetic material—wrapped in a protein coat. Measured in millionths of inches, it is virtually undetectable except under an electron microscope; taken into the human body, however, it is capable of enormous destructive power. The hepatitis virus migrates into the tissues of the liver; and because this site is particularly vulnerable to it, the virus is able to inject itself into a liver cell, where it swiftly takes control. Using the cell's own energy and materials, it begins to replicate. Between a hundred and a thousand new viruses can be produced within that single cell, each identical to the first invading virus. This newly made viral assault force soon bursts from the cell it has commandeered, destroying it, and spreads out in all directions to attack nearby cells. Within each of the newly invaded cells, the deadly process is repeated: a single invader uses the cell's own components to create more viruses, which then burst from the cell to attack others. Unchallenged, this invading force would, implacably and with exponentially increasing speed, destroy the cells of the liver and then the liver itself—and with it, the body.

But even as the replicated viruses burst from that first doomed liver cell, the body begins its counterattack.

Within the bloodstream, pulsing through the tissues that make up our skin, our muscles, and our internal organs, hundreds of millions of specialized cells—commonly known as white blood cells—are at work defending the body's territory. Like sentries, a special group of these cells, called *phagocytes,* are constantly alert to the presence of any foreign cells or cellular debris they may encounter in their repeated circuit of the body—anything not recognized as part of the body. When phagocytes, passing through the liver, encounter that first contingent of hepatitis viruses, their strategy is direct and effective. In an effort to kill the invader before it has a chance to multiply, they simply engulf and destroy the virus-infected cells. They literally "eat" the invading organisms (*phagocyte* means "cell eater").

In cell-to-cell combat, phagocytes are swift and efficient killers. But wave after wave of newly created viruses burst from the invaded liver cells; the enemy is multiplying too quickly. Phagocytes simply cannot keep up with the rapid destruction of the body's cells. And so a second line of defense, far more complex and powerful than phagocytes, is set in motion: a group of specialized white blood cells called *T lymphocytes.*

T lymphocytes, or T cells, have evolved the extraordinary ability to recognize the precise identity of a foreign cell or substance. Unlike phagocytes, which consume not only invading organisms but all sorts of cellular debris that washes into the bloodstream, T cells are specifically targeted to a particular organism or foreign substance. T cells not only recognize an invader, but the precise identity of the invader. They do so by identifying chemical markers carried on the membranes of virtually all living cells. These chemical substances play a variety of different roles in the functional life of microorganisms, among them one that is crucial to immune responses: each specific combination of chemical substances declares the uniqueness of the cell or virus that bears it. Circulating T cells have evolved the ability to recognize these unique chemical substances. Even more amazing, they have learned to distinguish between the cells that make up our own bodies and those that represent microorganisms which may invade the body and cause disease. It has been estimated that the immune system can recognize a million different molecules that identify cells or substances foreign to the body.

Through the major blood vessels, into the microscopic branchings of the capillaries, out into the arteries of the lymph system and then back again into major blood vessels, a specialized group of T cells called helper T cells circulate. Their cyclic journey takes them through virtually every tissue of the body. When circulating T cells genetically preprogrammed to recognize the hepatitis B virus come in contact with the invader, they immediately begin to reproduce. And a call—chemical signals released into the bloodstream—goes out for reinforcements. Additional phagocytes and T cells race to the site of infection to join the fight.

As they arrive, groups of helper T cells begin to leave the liver and make their way through the bloodstream. These T cells carry not only news of the battle, but the specific nature of the enemy at hand. Their destination: the nearest lymph nodes.

The lymph system mirrors the body's circulatory system, extending its branching vessels wherever the veins and arteries of the bloodstream are found. The lymph nodes placed along the lymph system represent small cell-manufacturing factories. With the arrival of T cells from the site of infection, two important mechanisms are set in motion within these cellular factories. First, helper T cells trigger the production of a new kind of T cell. These new T cells differ from helper T cells in one crucial way: they are designed for the sole purpose of attacking and killing the cells within the liver that have been infected by the hepatitis virus. These specialized T cells, called killer T cells, quickly spill into the bloodstream and travel to the site of infection to join the battle against the intruding virus. By killing virus-infected cells before the viruses can replicate, killer T cells play a critical role in blocking further spread of the infection.

Meanwhile, helper T cells in the lymph nodes have also made contact with another set of specialized blood cells, called *B lymphocytes*—and the second major activity of the lymph nodes begins.

B cells reside in the lymph nodes, awaiting only the arrival of helper T cells in order to begin their work. When T cells carrying information about the invading organism encounter B cells, they activate these cells to begin to reproduce. Newly created B cells in turn begin to manufacture chemical weapons, called *antibodies,* which are specifically engineered to destroy the invading hepatitis virus. The production of antibodies may take two or three days to reach effective levels. But once antibody molecules are released into the bloodstream, they surge toward the site of the infection, joining the killer T cells and phagocytes in their fight.

Killer T cells and antibodies are the immune system's most potent weapons. Programmed to target a specific virus and virus-infected cells, they attack and destroy the invaders before the viruses can replicate and inject themselves into other cells. Helper T cells continue to call in new recruits, as phagocytes, ranging over the site of the infection, engulf and destroy the debris of damaged cells and viral materials—the wreckage of battle. As the battle is won, a third population of T cells, called suppressor T cells, begin to release substances that slow down and finally halt the activities of the other immune cells.

In the aftermath of an immune response, one of the great marvels of the body's complex defense system comes into play. Large numbers of specialized T and B cells have been created during the body's struggle to defend itself: helper and killer T cells programmed to identify and attack cells infected by the hepatitis virus, and B cells programmed to produce antibodies specifically designed to neutralize that virus. After the infection subsides, large numbers of these specialized cells are still present in the bloodstream. And they will remain there, some for as long as twenty years. If a hepatitis B virus again invades the body, a year from now, or two, or twenty, these cells, called memory T and B cells, will act as an early warning system, rapidly producing killer T cells and antibodies, giving the body a head start it did not have in the first encounter with the invader. Memory T and B cells can bestow immunity to many diseases after a single exposure.

Only in recent years have we been able to piece together precise details of this extraordinary system of self-defense. And there is still much to discover. We are only beginning to understand the language of immune responses—those chemical signals and commands by which the cells of the immune system communicate with each other. Each cell of the immune system receives and transmits enormous amounts of information. Immune cells engage in something very much like conversation: an elaborate network of announcements, commands, and countercommands. The placement, the timing, and the nature of every signal is exquisitely precise; the effect of a single command extremely powerful. By deciphering the key words in this immunologic vocabulary, researchers have begun to gain important insights into the way the body defends itself against disease. And the future of immunology holds out a breathtaking possibility. By learning these key words, researchers may discover how to mimic the commands of the immune system, and use the language of immune responses to stimulate the immune system itself in the fight against disease.

Revolutionary new technologies such as recombinant DNA techniques are providing immunologists with unprecedented tools to make this possible. Today we are able to do what was previously unthinkable: to isolate individual genes and then move them from one organism to another, creating hybrid cells that did not previously exist in nature. We can literally design new cells engineered for our own purposes. Human hormones such as insulin are now routinely produced in large quantities simply by isolating and then moving the human gene for insulin production into bacteria that can be grown in large numbers. Immunologists have already begun using these techniques to create specialized cells that will produce the chemical products of the immune system. These chemicals, the first words that we have learned to speak in the immune system's language, are now being tested in experiments designed to control immune responses.

Recent insights into the form and function of the human immune system have also given immunologists new understanding of a wide range of diseases that have long baffled medical researchers, among them diseases of the immune system itself. The complex activity of phagocytes and T cells crucially depends on their ability to distinguish between the healthy cells of the body—that vast cellular network that is "self"—and damaged or disease-producing cells—anything that is "non-self." In a category of diseases called *autoimmune disorders,* the body loses its ability to distinguish between self and non-self. The immune system literally turns on the body, rejecting healthy cells as if they were invaders. In Goodpasture's syndrome, for example, the immune system loses its ability to recognize the cells of the kidney as self. Wave after wave of immune cells attack the kidneys, ultimately destroying them as ruthlessly as if they were some life-threatening virus. We do not fully understand what causes the immune system's fatal error in recognition. But we have begun to recognize that a number of once mysterious diseases of unknown origin are, in fact, autoimmune disorders—rheumatoid arthritis, for example, and the central nervous system disorder of multiple sclerosis, as well as myasthenia gravis and systemic lupus erythematosus.

In certain circumstances, the normal functioning of immune

responses can prove just as deadly as autoimmune rejection. When a donor heart, kidney, or liver is transplanted into the body, for example, the immune system quite accurately recognizes the cells of the new organ as foreign invaders. Imagining the body to be under attack, the system begins to mount a swift and furious counterattack on the foreign cells, destroying them and ultimately rejecting the transplant—literally killing it within the body. The phenomenon of rejection remains the most serious problem facing surgical transplantation. At present, physicians are able to control the rejection mechanism only by administering drugs that suppress the immune system itself. These immunosuppressive drugs are nonspecific; they suppress the entire spectrum of immune responses, leaving the body prey to a host of infectious agents, some of them life-threatening. But as immunologists begin to decipher the signals that determine "self" and "non-self," we will discover ways to use the immune system's own language to trick the body into accepting specific donor tissue. That breakthrough, when it comes, may offer new forms of treatment for autoimmune disorders as well.

The latest insights of modern immunology have also begun to illuminate one of the oldest medical mysteries—the nature of allergy and asthma. Only in this century have we begun to understand that allergic reactions are immune responses to inert foreign substances taken into the body. Today, immunologists have discovered the intricate chemical signals that link a grain of pollen to the wheezing, itchy eyes, and runny, congested nose of hay fever. By blocking one or more of those chemical signals, researchers hope to control the body's immune response to pollen, bee stings, and other allergens.

The human immune system is at work in our defense even

before the moment of birth. Indeed, insights into the complex immunologic relationship of mother and fetus are among the most fascinating discoveries of modern immunology. A mother and the child forming within her womb are locked in a fierce struggle for survival. Even as the mother's body nurtures and provides for the fetus, the maternal immune system, recognizing this new life as foreign, seeks to destroy it. The fetus and the placenta that protects it have evolved a special arsenal of defense mechanisms to elude and subvert the constant threat of attack by the mother's immune cells. The discovery and understanding of these mechanisms have led researchers to new insights into the causes of certain reproductive disorders—infertility, for example, as well as some of the diseases of pregnancy. Immunologic breakthroughs in reproductive immunology may well result in a new, safer, method of contraception: a contraceptive "vaccine."

Paradoxically, our newest insights into the way life begins may also provide answers to the mystery of one of the leading causes of death: cancer. Immunologists have begun to realize that the strategies a fetus uses to defend itself from the mother's immune system are, in many ways, the same strategies a tumor uses to escape detection and destruction within the body. The immune system possesses the ability to detect cancer cells as invaders and to move against them with a full arsenal of cellular weapons. And yet for reasons that have never been clearly understood, the body's surveillance against cancer cells can sometimes break down. By understanding how and why tumor cells manage to survive despite the powerful defenses of the body, researchers hope to find the key to a cure for cancer itself.

Immunologists have also begun to investigate the relationship of the immune system to other systems such as the nervous and endocrine systems of the body. Recent research has provided fascinating evidence of the effect of stress in suppressing immune responsiveness, for example, and of the mechanisms by which exercise may help enhance the activities of the immune system. These findings have given us a renewed sense of the wonder of the human body as a whole, of many complex systems interrelated and interdependent.

Cancer research, the study of autoimmune diseases, and the demands of transplant surgery have each brought a new urgency to the study of immune responses. But no single event has so galvanized immunologic research as the unprecedented appearance, in 1979, of a new and lethal disease: Acquired Immune Deficiency Syndrome, or AIDS. Victims of the disease manifest a puzzling array of previously obscure diseases: rare cancers, a lethal form of pneumonia, and other uncommon and life-threatening infections. It is now clear that these diseases are no more than symptoms of a single underlying disease: the nearly complete breakdown of the immune system itself. By studying the profound breakdown of immune responses in AIDS patients, researchers have already gained new insights into the basic functioning of this system—insights which may eventually offer treatment and a cure for AIDS as well as other immune deficiency diseases.

Immunology is a young science. During its brief history, breakthroughs in understanding have often raised more questions than they have answered. The fundamental mechanisms of immune responses have remained baffling mysteries despite the best efforts of brilliant investigators. But in the last ten years, a virtual explosion in research and understanding has taken place. Scientists have watched with growing excitement as a number of diverse research fields have begun to converge on the study of the human immune system. Today, immunology represents the great new frontier of medical research.

This book is an attempt to chart that new and exciting terrain. The first chapters explore the latest breakthroughs in our understanding of the form and function of the human immune system. The last chapters of the book will explore how these breakthroughs offer new insight into physiologic processes that have long baffled medical researchers. While every effort has been made to present the most recent research, progress in the field of immunology is taking place so rapidly that new and important findings are announced at an accelerating rate. These findings will no doubt affect some of the information presented here. But even the most revolutionary discoveries grow out of research that has gone before. This book should provide a useful foundation for understanding the breakthroughs that will almost certainly expand our knowledge of the nature and function of the human immune system in the coming years.

Perhaps the best way to begin to grasp the awesome power and complexity of the body's defense system is to understand the varied, shifting, and insidious nature of the opposing force —bacteria, viruses, protozoa, and the other agents of disease.

two

THE ENEMIES

Nature abounds with little round things.

LEWIS THOMAS, 1971

The scientific method was simple and straightforward. Once he had perfected the design of his microscope, Anton van Leeuwenhoek set out with almost childlike curiosity to examine and record the world that existed beyond the range of his naked eye. In one of his experiments, he scraped material from his teeth, added a drop of rainwater, and then placed the concoction under his handmade lens. "I then saw, with great wonder," he wrote in a letter to the Royal Society of London in 1683, "that in the said matter there were many very little animalcules, very prettily a-moving."* Of these tiny creatures,

*Dubois, R., M. Pines, and the Editors of Time-Life Books. 1980. *Health & Disease.* Alexandria, VA.: Time-Life Books.

some "shot through the water like a pike," others "spun round like a top," and still others "went ahead so nimbly, and hovered so together that you might imagine them to be a big swarm of gnats or flies."

Leeuwenhoek's seventeenth-century discovery, though less embattled, was no less revolutionary than the Copernican claim that the sun and not the earth stood at the center of the planetary system. For in that first glimpse of life through the handmade lens of an early microscope, Leeuwenhoek had seen that we share not only the world but ourselves, our own bodies, with a host of creatures invisible to the unaided eye.

More than a hundred years passed before scientists looked again with much interest at these tiny creatures, and another fifty after that before Louis Pasteur made a startling pronouncement. Pasteur had come to recognize, by 1857, that microbes—Leeuwenhoek's "very little animalcules"—were more than just cohabitants in our world. Certain of them appeared to be responsible for turning milk sour, others for fermenting wine. Still others, he believed, were very likely the agents of disease.

With Pasteur's discovery, scientists had at last recognized the enemy. And the ancient battle against disease became a modern science.

Returning again and again to the shooting, spinning, hovering creatures he had glimpsed in the milky field of his microscope, Leeuwenhoek patiently sketched diagrams to record the microscopic organisms he had discovered. As an indication of scale, he compared their size to common objects—grains of sand, for example, and mustard seeds. His drawings were painstaking and sharply detailed—so accurate, in fact, that a microbiologist looking at them today would recognize exactly what Leeuwenhoek had seen: bacteria, protozoa, and yeast.

Under a light microscope, bacteria appear as slender rods or clusters of round cells. Most of them measure only a few thousandths of a millimeter in length or diameter. Their small size and relative simplicity belie their extraordinary power. Bacteria have caused some of the deadliest plagues in history.

The bacterium *Yersinia pestis,* spreading bubonic plague across Europe in the fourteenth century, killed more than twenty-five million people—one-fourth of the European population. *Yersinia pestis* struck again in 1664, killing more than 70,000 people—one out of every five—during the Great Plague of London. And as late as 1894, an epidemic of bubonic plague killed 100,000 people in Canton and Hong Kong before spreading out along shipping channels to cause ten million deaths worldwide.

Other bacterial infections have been nearly as lethal. The nineteenth century saw successive waves of a terrifyingly swift and deadly disease sweep across large parts of the world. A person waking up in apparently good health, struck by the disease, might be dead and buried by evening. The disease was cholera, the silent killer a bacterium called *Vibrio cholerae,* transmitted through water and food contaminated by raw sewage.

We now know that bacteria are single-celled organisms, alive and fully capable of generating the energy and chemical substances they need to maintain and reproduce themselves. They are self-sufficient and, because of their relative simplicity, remarkably hardy, able to survive in extremes of both pressure and temperature. Bacteria have been found in ocean depths of seven miles and at atmospheric heights of more than forty miles, surviving in hot springs as well as the polar ice caps.

Like all living cells, a bacterial cell contains genetic material. The single strand of deoxyribonucleic acid (DNA) within a bacterial cell contains the blueprint for producing at least a thousand different proteins—all of the information necessary for creating a new bacterium. A nutrient broth surrounds the DNA, containing the molecules and machinery necessary for the normal function of the cell. The cell itself is bounded by a multilayered membrane. Whatever chemicals bacteria may require but cannot produce must be transferred from the external environment across this cell membrane.

Bacteria are the cause of a wide range of human diseases—rheumatic fever, typhoid, dysentery, tuberculosis, leprosy, syphilis, anthrax, diphtheria, cholera, and tetanus among them. In virtually all cases, bacteria attack the body by producing powerful toxins—chemicals that can damage specific tissues and cells, block the normal function of important substances in the blood and tissues, or interfere with the various regulatory systems that control the movement of fluids between the blood and tissues. One group of toxins, called *exotoxins,* are produced within the bacterial cell and then secreted through the cell membrane into the surrounding tissue, where the damage they cause can be lethal.

The cholera bacterium, *Vibrio cholerae,* for example, kills by producing powerful exotoxins that attack the cells lining the small intestine that are responsible for the regulation of water and salt balance. The result is severe diarrhea and dehydration. *Corynebacterium diphtheriae,* the causative agent of diphtheria, produces an exotoxin that not only destroys nearby cells but travels through the bloodstream to destroy the tissues of distant organs—primarily the heart and kidneys. But of all bacterial exotoxins, those produced by *Clostridium botulinum*—the causative agent of botulism—are the most potent. Almost as soon as these bacteria are ingested, they begin to release exotoxins that block the transmission of nerve impulses at the junction between nerves and muscle cells. Vision becomes distorted and breathing difficult, and the victim experiences muscular weakness. In more than half of all cases of botulism, death follows from paralysis of the respiratory center. The toxins of *Clostridium botulinum* are so potent that as little as 0.000036 ounce of the toxin would be enough to kill one million laboratory guinea pigs.

Recently, exotoxins were also implicated in the appearance of a new and mysterious disease syndrome. In 1978, an alarming number of women between the ages of twelve and fifty-two began to exhibit symptoms of fever, rash, diarrhea, vomiting, and a severe drop in blood pressure—symptoms usually associated with some form of bacteria-induced shock. By 1980, some 300 cases of the puzzling syndrome had been reported, twenty-five of them fatal. Researchers finally implicated certain brands of highly absorbent tampons, apparently responsible for a severe *Staphylococcus aureus* infection in the vagina. These bacteria, it was found, secrete a highly toxic substance called enterotoxin F. By poisoning nearby cells, this toxin produces the array of symptoms of toxic shock syndrome. The same toxin may play a role in other forms of *S. aureus* infections, in men as well as women.

Exotoxins destroy by directly attacking specific tissues and organs in the body. Another group of bacterial toxins wreaks havoc in more subtle, devious ways—by releasing substances called *endotoxins,* which act indirectly by generating an exaggerated and potentially lethal response from the cells of the body's immune system. Released from the cell walls of bacteria, endotoxins can cause certain immune cells to release substances that trigger a drop in blood pressure, induce fever and chills, and in extreme cases cause substantial organ damage. Endotoxins can trigger the production of antibodies—not only antibodies specific to the invader, but every antibody that the immune system can produce, including relatively rare but highly destructive *autoantibodies,* which attack the body's own cells. In a growing chain reaction, antibodies activate substances in the blood that contribute to widespread tissue damage. The immune system's uncontrolled response to endotoxins makes them both extremely powerful and highly destructive. A laboratory mouse injected with endotoxin will be dead within two hours, of complete respiratory and cardiovascular collapse. Endotoxin-producing bacteria are responsible for a variety of serious diseases, including typhoid and dysentery.

In addition to exotoxins and endotoxins, bacteria possess a third deadly weapon, a group of substances called *impedins* or *aggressins,* which can directly subvert the immune system and other functions of the body. No other disease agent produces so many of these potent substances as the bacterium *Staphylococcus aureus. S. aureus* releases *coagulase,* an impedin that causes the formation of blood clots that effectively block the movement of phagocytes and other immune cells to the site of infection. *S. aureus* also releases at least three impedins that can block the ability of phagocytes to engulf and destroy it, as well as a powerful impedin that can actually kill phagocytes. Other bacterial species secrete similar impedins, including one that can break up and neutralize antibody molecules targeted to destroy the invading bacteria.

Paradoxically, for all their power to destroy life, bacteria are crucial to our survival. The soil contains large numbers of bacteria which, through their special ability to metabolize chemicals, are able to break down the tissues of dead plants and animals, recycling the basic components of life. Like all animals, we ourselves provide a nutrient-rich environment for bacteria. Millions of bacteria exist on the surface of the skin, in the mouth, within the respiratory tract. Even greater numbers reside in the small and large intestines, breaking down the food we eat into usable compounds. These benign bacteria, referred to as the *normal flora,* are essential to human life, and we exist with them in a delicate symbiotic relationship.

The nature of bacteria as both friend and foe makes the job of immune defense extraordinarily difficult. In order to defend the body, the cells of the immune system must first be able to spot the enemy. They must be able to distinguish between the body's own cells and invading *pathogens*—the agents of disease. But more than that, they must be able to distinguish between pathogens and the normal flora, allowing acceptable levels of the normal flora to exist while at the same time completely eradicating infectious organisms. To meet this challenge, cells of the immune system have evolved the ability to recognize and identify an enormous number of different cells and substances.

Every bacterium—indeed, virtually every living cell—bears on its cell wall a group of identifying molecules that are characteristic of that particular cell species. These molecules, usually made up of proteins and carbohydrates, are like the fingerprint of the cell, identifying it and distinguishing it from other types of cells. One unique set of molecules, for example, declares its bearer to be the bacterium *Escherichia coli;* another set identifies *Streptococcus pyogenes;* a slightly different set announces *Vibrio cholerae.* Because the identifying molecules of bacterial cells are different in their arrangement from the proteins and carbohydrates on the surface of human cells, the immune system can recognize them as foreign, or "non-self." Such foreign molecules—molecules which will trigger the immune system to respond in a profound and determined way against them—are called *antigens.* The immune system detects the presence of its enemies by way of these antigens. And at the moment an immune cell detects a foreign antigen, it sets in motion a complex chain reaction designed to destroy the invader and protect the body from subsequent attack.

Of the body's cellular enemies, bacteria were the first identified and are today the most thoroughly understood. Most of the mechanisms of bacterial infection are well known to us, and the treatment and control of most bacterial diseases are within our grasp. But another of the body's implacable enemies, the virus, has guarded its secrets more zealously.

In 1885, Louis Pasteur set out to isolate the disease organism that caused rabies—an agent we now know to be a virus. In early experiments, he passed the saliva of a rabid dog through a cloth filter fine enough to isolate bacterial microbes. But when he examined the residue in the filter, he could find no microorganisms. And yet when the same saliva was injected into a test animal, it invariably caused rabies. What was this unseen agent that caused such destruction?

Pasteur tried other experiments. He found that if he first allowed the saliva from a rabid dog to dry on a microscope slide and then injected it into a test animal, the saliva was no longer infectious. Whatever had once caused the disease was now gone—either removed or killed by the drying process. Pasteur then began to experiment with the spinal cords of rabid animals. These, too, appeared to contain the mysterious pathogen. And when the spinal tissues were dried and injected, they too failed to transmit the disease. Pasteur already knew that he could protect sheep or cows against anthrax by killing anthrax bacteria and then injecting the dead bacterial cells into the animals. Now he tried the same experiment with rabies. He injected the dried spinal tissue from rabid animals into healthy test animals. When he later attempted to infect the test animals with rabies, he discovered that the animals were immune to the disease.

Pasteur had failed to isolate the pathogen that caused rabies, but by discovering an effective vaccine for rabies, he had achieved an important breakthrough, one that very quickly began to save human lives.

Pasteur's rabies vaccine was not the first successful vaccine, however. Indeed, the history of attempts at vaccination goes back to ancient times. The people of ancient China and western Asia had observed that individuals who contracted smallpox were resistant to a second attack, and primitive attempts were made to immunize people against severe smallpox infection by inoculating them with fluid obtained from people with mild cases of the disease.

It was not until 1721 that the practice of immunization came to Europe, when Lady Mary Wortley Montagu, wife of the British Ambassador to Turkey, returned to England and had her daughter immunized against smallpox, repeating a procedure that had been performed on her son three years earlier. Of the procedure she wrote:

> The small-pox, so fatal, and so general amongst us, is here entirely harmless. . . . People send to one another to know if any of their family has a mind to have the small-pox: they make parties for this purpose, and when they are met (commonly fifteen or sixteen together), the old woman comes with a nutshell of the matter of the best sort of small-pox, and asks what vein you please to have opened. She immediately rips open that you offer her, with a large needle (which gives you no more pain than a common scratch) and puts into the vein, as much matter as can lie upon the head of a needle. . . . There is no example of anyone that had died in it: and you may believe I am well satisfied of the safety of this experiment, since I intend to try it on my dear little son. I am patriot enough to take pains to bring this useful invention into fashion in England.*

Unfortunately, this particular procedure of immunization—called *variolation*—was not always successful. In some cases, instead of producing a mild case of the disease, variolation actually caused a full-scale infection of smallpox. In other cases, the inoculating fluid, contaminated with other organisms, infected the patient with diseases like leprosy or syphilis.

More than fifty years after Lady Montagu imported variolation to England, an English physician named Edward Jenner produced the first fully effective and safe vaccination against smallpox. Curiously, Jenner himself never understood the fundamental relationship of disease and vaccination. Like Pasteur, he never glimpsed the organisms that caused the disease. He simply observed that people who developed cowpox, a mild disease that resembled smallpox, seemed to be protected from contracting the far more serious illness. By inoculating people with cowpox, Jenner discovered, he could protect them from the ravages of smallpox. The method worked; no one knew

*Barrett, J. T. 1983. *Textbook of Immunology: An Introduction to Immunochemistry and Immunology.* St. Louis: C. V. Mosby Co. Quoted from: Dixon, C. W. 1962. *Smallpox.* London: J. & A. Churchill, Ltd.

why. Indeed, for almost a century, the exact nature of the organism that caused the disease would remain a baffling mystery.

Pasteur's rabies vaccine in 1885 was an important breakthrough because he had managed to develop a vaccine by intentionally weakening, or *attenuating,* the unseen agent that caused the disease. In the years that followed, researchers tried to apply Pasteur's method in the fight against other diseases like polio, measles, yellow fever, and rubella. But their attempts, in most cases, were met with puzzling failures. For no matter what they tried—chemicals, extreme heat, or poisons—scientists were unable to duplicate Pasteur's success. They could not seem to weaken or kill the disease agent and at the same time preserve its ability to produce immunity against a subsequent infection. The unseen pathogen remained a mystery.

It was not until the invention of the electron microscope that researchers at last began to fully understand the mystery of the virus. The electron microscope vastly extended the range of our vision into the microcosm of cells and molecules. Single cells could be magnified as much as 500,000 times. With this new power of vision, researchers glimpsed for the first time the agent for viral infection. Suddenly it was clear why Pasteur had been unable to isolate the rabies pathogen in a fine cloth filter. Under the electron microscope, viruses were small, dark strands that measured no more than one one-hundred-thousandth of an inch—far smaller and less complex than bacterial cells. Indeed, ten million virus particles could be placed on the head of a pin. In Pasteur's experiment, the rabies virus had passed easily through the cloth filter, remaining in the specimen to infect again.

But with one mystery solved, another quickly took its place. For when researchers now attempted to grow viruses in culture, they were again frustrated by failure. They used techniques developed in bacterial research, placing viruses in the same nutrient solution that allowed bacteria to grow. Nothing happened. The viruses remained inert, lifeless; for all that anyone knew of life and death, these viruses were dead. Yet the same viruses, injected into laboratory animals, seemed suddenly to come alive, reproducing themselves, triggering disease. Why?

The solution came with another technological breakthrough—the ability to maintain living cells outside the body. By a laborious process of trial and error, researchers developed an artificial culture medium in which, for the first time, living animal tissue could be kept alive outside the body. When a small number of viruses were introduced into the cells of this tissue, the viruses began to reproduce. Using tissue cultures, investigators were now able to grow large numbers of viruses for study. And under the electron microscope, they could actually see the process by which viruses apparently came to life. With that, the great central mystery of the virus was solved.

Viruses, we now know, stand on the line between living and nonliving matter. An isolated virus is, to all extents and purposes, dead. It cannot grow; it cannot reproduce itself; under a microscope it appears completely inert. But when a virus comes in contact with a living host cell, a series of chemical reactions take place which allow the virus to move into the cell. Once there, the virus commandeers the cell's machinery and adapts it to its own purposes, instructing the cell to create the components needed for viral replication.

The fundamental simplicity of a virus allows it to occupy its unique place on the boundary between living and nonliving. In its simplest form, a virus is nothing more than an inner core of material that contains the genetic information for reproduction, and an outer covering of protein. Certain viruses also bear an outer envelope derived from the host cell. And that is all. Unlike a bacterium, a virus contains neither the materials nor the mechanisms for growth, reproduction, or movement. Its inner core of genetic material—either ribonucleic acid (RNA) or deoxyribonucleic acid (DNA)—contains only the *instructions* for viral reproduction. Once inside a host cell, the viral genetic material takes over the synthesizing machinery and materials of the cell itself.

Before it can invade a host cell, however, a virus must first attach itself to a specific site on the surface of the cell, called a *viral recognition site.* If the cell does not have this specific site, then the virus simply cannot inject itself. That cell is resistant to attack. Different cells of the body appear to possess different viral recognition sites. Nervous tissue, for example, possesses recognition sites for rabies virus but not the hepatitis virus. This requirement for specific viral recognition sites may explain why certain organs and tissues of the body are more susceptible to one virus than another.

Once it binds to a viral recognition site, a series of chemical reactions moves the virus into the cell through the cell membrane. Stripping down to the central core of genetic material, the virus then begins to use the cell's energy and constituents to produce large amounts of genetic material and viral protein. From these raw materials, new viruses are assembled. The newly formed viruses may then leave the invaded cell by *budding off,* retracing the steps they took to enter the cell—wrapping themselves in a small part of the cell membrane and then separating. Or the newly made viruses may simply cause the invaded cell to burst, releasing them and destroying the cell. Between a hundred and a thousand viruses can be reproduced in a single infected cell. Released, these viruses fan out to invade nearby cells—and the process of injection, replication, and dissemination is repeated.

In most instances of viral invasion, the resulting infection is acute. The disease agents are detected; the immune system responds by attacking and destroying the infected cells as well as invading viruses; and after the infection has been resolved, specialized immune cells confer permanent immunity or resistance to the particular species of virus that has invaded. The success of vaccination depends on this sequence of events. Jenner's vaccine against smallpox worked simply because the body's immune system worked. When Jenner injected cowpox into the body, this rather mild disease ran its course. After the immune system mounted a successful counterattack against the virus, large numbers of the long-lived immune cells called memory cells began to circulate, alert to the specific surface antigens of the cowpox virus. By a simple stroke of good fortune, it happens that the surface antigens of the cowpox virus are almost identical to those of the smallpox virus—so close, in fact, that the immune system cannot tell them apart. If the far more dangerous smallpox virus invaded after vaccination with cowpox, the body was already prepared to produce the proper antibodies and immune cells that could effectively fight the new invader.

Pasteur's rabies vaccine worked in much the same way. By drying the saliva or brain tissue of rabid animals, he seriously weakened the power of the viruses contained within it. When these attenuated viruses were then injected into the body, they began the process of infection—but much more slowly, and with far less virulence. The immune system, sensing the invaders, immediately began producing active immune cells and antibodies. Pasteur's method had given the body a crucial advantage. The immune system could mount its defense before the weakened viruses could gain a foothold. And after the viruses were destroyed, circulating memory cells retained the ability to defend the body again and again against other invasions of the rabies virus.

The theory and method of all vaccines are basically the same: by injecting either attenuated or inactivated viruses into the body, the immune system is triggered to respond. But because the injected viruses are weakened or inactive, they pose no real danger. Once circulating antibodies and long-lived memory cells are produced against the specific virus, the body is immune to subsequent attack.

As simple as the theory of vaccination is, the development of vaccines for specific diseases has been a long, slow, and frustrating process—as the researchers who tried to follow Pasteur's success discovered. After the development of the rabies vaccine, forty years would pass before the next milestone in immunization—the achievement of vaccines against diphtheria and tetanus in 1925—and another thirty before researchers managed to develop a vaccine against polio. The problem was frustratingly simple. To create a safe and reliable vaccine, researchers had to find a way to weaken the strength of a particular virus without altering the ability of the immune system to recognize the protein antigens that surround the viral genetic material. In most attempts, unfortunately, weakening the virus disturbed the arrangement of the antigen molecules to such a degree that the immune response to the *altered* viral antigens did not extend to the antigens as they normally exist on the virus. Researchers have discovered that the antigens of each species of virus have their own unique set of properties. Some are destroyed by exposure to air, for example, while others are not. Some can be attenuated by exposure to elevated temperatures, while others show no sensitivity to temperature at all. Certain chemicals affect some viruses, while others remain unaffected. The search for methods to weaken the strength of a specific virus without severely modifying its antigens has been one of trial and error. And for a number of viruses, that search continues.

The full force of the body's defense against viral invasion begins as soon as a virus invades a cell. As the virus commandeers the machinery of the invaded cell, it sets in motion a process that places viral antigens on the surface of the cell, signaling the body that the enemy is present. But a number of viruses have evolved a clever way to elude the body's immune surveillance system. The herpes simplex type 1 virus, for example, is able to survive within an infected cell for prolonged periods without bringing about the cell's destruction. As a result, these viruses can exist within the body for long periods of time without being detected by the immune system. After causing primary lesions of the skin, the mouth, the eyes, or the brain, herpes simplex type 1 will retreat to the nerve cells that make contact with the area of the original infection. By entering a nerve cell, the virus is able literally to hide out, protected from the attack of immune cells. After a period of latency, the viruses can make their way back to the site of infection and once again induce lesions. Then, before the immune system can marshal its forces, the herpes simplex type 1 virus simply retreats again to the safety of the nerve cells. This pattern of attack and retreat can be repeated indefinitely, causing the repeated flare-ups associated with herpes infection. Scientists do not know exactly how the herpes virus accomplishes its strategy. The nature of the events that trigger the recurrence of herpes infection aren't clearly understood either, although it has been established that the reactivation of the virus often occurs after emotional stress, menstruation, or fever.

Most of us carry latent viruses within us. Epstein-Barr virus —associated with infectious mononucleosis and Burkitt's lymphoma, a tumor of the white blood cells—can be found in almost 80 percent of the U.S. population. More than half of all Americans between the ages of eighteen and twenty-five, and over 80 percent of those over thirty-five, exhibit evidence of having been infected by cytomegalovirus, a virus which characteristically remains latent in the body for long periods. When activated, cytomegalovirus can produce a form of skin rash, hepatitis, or a mononucleosis-like syndrome in adults. In its most dangerous form, latent cytomegalovirus can cause severe birth defects in the children of virally infected mothers. In a number of confirmed cases, reactivation of the virus during pregnancy has led to the infection of the fetus. Ten percent of infants infected in utero with cytomegalovirus are born with congenital defects, including mental retardation. And one hospital study in Rochester, New York revealed that the I.Q. scores of infants born with the infection were significantly lower than the average scores for a control group of healthy infants. Cytomegalovirus may well be the most common viral cause of mental retardation.

One group of viruses, called *slow viruses,* have latency periods that may last for several years. The slow virus that causes a rare disease called kuru, for example, can remain latent in the body for up to five years before causing the symptoms of disease. Kuru is a degenerative disease of the central nervous system characterized by uncoordinated movements, mental deterioration, and tremors. Death usually occurs about a year after the onset of these symptoms. The disease was first observed in a single tribe in New Guinea, where it most often affected women and children. Epidemiological studies of the tribe implicated a bizarre tribal practice: by tradition, members of the tribe consumed the brains of the dead. Women were most often involved in the preparation of the ritual feast. Researchers injected brain tissue from human kuru victims into chimpanzees, and within a period of five years the animals developed a similar disease. It is now believed that the virus was transmitted by direct contact between the hands of the tribal women and the brain tissue of dead kuru victims. With the outlawing of cannibalism, the disease has disappeared.

We do not yet understand the mechanisms by which a latent virus, dormant within the body for long periods, comes suddenly and destructively alive. Reactivation may result from some change in the body's internal environment, or perhaps a change in the virus itself. Viruses are known to undergo genetic changes, or *mutations,* which may alter their behavior within the body. Most often, these genetic mutations will change the antigens on the viral surface—that group of substances that declare what and who the virus is.

The influenza virus is among the most changeable. Periodically, influenza viruses undergo major genetic mutations that can result in new viral strains with altered surface antigens. Memory cells, alert to the presence of antigen markers of a previous influenza virus, may be blind to the new, altered form.

The genetic variability of the influenza virus gives it a dangerous advantage: it can alter its antigenic identity and strike again with the virulence of a completely new disease. Sudden appearances of new influenza strains have resulted in many explosive epidemics worldwide. One of the most devastating outbreaks of any infectious disease in recorded history, in fact, was the 1918–1919 pandemic of "Spanish flu," a new, mutated strain of influenza that killed close to twenty-one million people. In 1957–1958, "Asian flu," another mutated strain of the influenza virus, resulted in seventy thousand deaths worldwide. The "Hong Kong flu" of 1968–1969 killed another thirty thousand.

Viewed under an electron microscope, the influenza virus is spherical, marked by characteristic surface projections. Changes in the chemical makeup of these surface projections often signal the appearance of a new, variant strain of the disease. When an outbreak of influenza occurred among U.S. Army recruits at Fort Dix, New Jersey in 1976, researchers quickly isolated the virus and examined its surface structure. They were alarmed to discover that the surface of this new, variant virus closely resembled the surface of the 1918 swine strain of influenza—the strain that had caused the devastating pandemic of "Spanish flu." This new virus (A/New Jersey/76) represented a major antigenic shift from the influenza viruses that had caused the 1968 epidemic (A/Hong Kong/68) and the 1975 epidemic (A/Victoria/75). Immunity to those earlier strains, with their different surface antigens, would not extend to this new variant.

Fearing a widespread epidemic, federal health officials initiated an unprecedented $135 million program to vaccinate the general public against the new virus. More than thirty-five million people received the vaccine as part of the National Influenza Immunization Program. When a small number of people developed serious paralysis after vaccination (for reasons that aren't clearly understood), the program was quickly halted. Ironically, only a few cases of A/New Jersey/76 influenza were ever confirmed. The virus may well have undergone another mutation, altering its surface antigens and reducing its virulence. The genetic variability of viruses like influenza is, at the most basic level, a tactic for survival. By periodically altering its identity, a virus can confound not only the body's immune system, but also our best efforts at creating a useful vaccine.

In recent years, researchers have discovered yet another trait of invading viruses—and a tactic that can prove deadly for the host organism. Instead of simply invading a cell and taking control of its DNA, a number of viruses—the Epstein-Barr virus and the herpes simplex type 2 virus among them—can actually incorporate their own genetic material into the DNA of the invaded cell. Although the total amount of incorporated viral DNA may be quite small compared to the host cell's DNA, it can induce a profound change in the life of the infected cell. For example, when a single gene along the strand of viral DNA, called an *oncogene,* is injected into the host DNA, it can transform the normal cell into a cancer cell. Unlike a normal cell, which contains built-in genetic controls on its own replication, a transformed cell can reproduce explosively and uncontrollably, divorcing itself from its genetic past and the body that originally nurtured it.

In addition to the herpes simplex and Epstein-Barr viruses, a number of other viruses have shown themselves to be oncogenic—cancer causing—in laboratory mice, rats, or guinea pigs. But although there are several likely candidates for human cancer viruses, investigators have yet to establish a definite link between a virus and cancer in humans. Still, there is no question that, at least in the test tube, certain viruses can cause normal cells to become cancerous.

Bacteria and viruses account for most of the common diseases found in the United States and other industrialized countries. But several of the most prevalent diseases worldwide are caused not by bacteria or viruses, but by single-celled organisms called protozoa. Malaria infects approximately 150 million people every year—the equivalent of almost three-quarters of the U.S. population. In Africa, malaria accounts for a startling 15 percent of all clinical illnesses. The disease, once thought to be transmitted by contaminated air arising from swamps and marshlands ("malaria" means "bad air" in Italian), is in fact caused by a group of protozoa classified under the genus *Plasmodium.* These single-celled parasites, like many protozoa, exist in a complex life cycle that includes both insect and human hosts. When the female anopheles mosquito bites a human infected with malaria, one form of *Plasmodium* passes into the mosquito's stomach. There the parasite matures, finally penetrating the stomach wall and migrating to the salivary glands. When the mosquito bites a second, uninfected individual, the malarial parasites pass into the human bloodstream and move quickly into the liver. There they begin to reproduce. Later, the parasites can return to the bloodstream, where they invade red blood cells and continue to reproduce, eventually rupturing the cells and causing anemia. Chills, high fever, and profuse sweating may flare up periodically. In many cases, the disease subsides, only to reappear—sometimes as much as a year later. Malaria may become chronic in some individuals; in others, untreated malaria can progress to high fever, delirium, and death.

Another protozoal infection, amoebic dysentery, is even more prevalent than malaria. The protozoan *Entamoeba histolytica,* which resides in the intestinal wall of its infected human host, is believed to infect up to 80 percent of the population in some tropical areas. Even in the United States, where sanitation measures largely prevent the spread of the parasite, between 1 and 5 percent of the population carries *E. histolytica.* The organism is transmitted primarily through the ingestion of contaminated water or food, although *E. histolytica* can also be spread through certain forms of sexual contact. Indeed, infections of *E. histolytica* as well as several other protozoa have become epidemic in a number of American cities in recent years, each transmitted by sexual contact. While most of the individuals infected with *E. histolytica* remain asymptomatic, 10 percent of its human hosts will exhibit bloody stools, indicating that the parasites have invaded the lining of the intestines. Bacterial infections often develop in the resulting ulcers. And in some cases, the parasite may move into the bloodstream to attack the liver and lungs.

E. histolytica, like several intestinal protozoa, can exist in a dormant state as a *parasitic cyst.* These cysts are extremely hardy and can survive for long periods of time outside the body —usually in contaminated soil, water, or food. Once ingested, however, they grow into mature, pathogenic protozoa. In healthy individuals, the immune system keeps the population of intestinal parasites under control. But when the immune system is compromised—primarily in malnourished infants and children—intestinal parasites can contribute as a cause of death.

In rare cases, the immune system's response to protozoa can be subverted by the parasites themselves. Protozoa of the genus *Trypanosoma*—the causative agents of African Sleeping Sickness and Chagas' disease—have evolved a devious strategy for eluding the body's immune surveillance system. These organisms are genetically programmed to alter their surface antigens periodically. Each time the body's immune cells target one set of antigens for destruction, the *Trypanosoma* alters the antigens. By doing so it disappears from view of the immune system until another set of immune cells, programmed to detect the new surface antigens, spots the altered parasite. Once again the immune system marshals its forces; but before the response can reach effective levels, *Trypanosoma* again shifts its surface antigens, continuing its existence in the midst of an active immune response against it.

In most cases, however, the immune system successfully controls most protozoal infections. We now know that a number of potentially lethal protozoa are quite common in the human body. As long as the immune system controls their growth, they pose no threat to life. But if the immune system becomes disabled, either through disease or the use of certain immunosuppressive drugs, these same protozoa can result in fatal infections. The protozoan *Pneumocystis carinii,* for example, resides in most of us. But among patients with Acquired Immune Deficiency Syndrome, whose immune systems are severely compromised, *Pneumocystis* is responsible for a lethal form of pneumonia. This form of pneumonia also strikes premature, malnourished, or debilitated infants—all of whom lack an active immune system. The mortality rates among such infants is sometimes as high as 50 percent.

Like *Pneumocystis carinii,* the protozoan *Toxoplasma gondii* is also commonly found in humans. Studies have shown that more than half of all adults in the U.S. are infected, and in certain subpopulations, that number may be as high as 80 percent. In healthy adults, the immune system successfully controls the growth of *Toxoplasma.* But in AIDS patients, in debilitated infants, and in individuals undergoing immunosuppressive drug therapy for malignancies or organ transplants, *Toxoplasma* can cause toxoplasmosis—a severe and life-threatening infection of the central nervous system. When this parasite invades the placenta and infects a fetus, it can lead to mental retardation or blindness.

Protozoa are not the only parasitic organisms to reside in a human host, feeding off the body's nutrients. *Helminths* (from the Greek word *helmins,* which means worm) represent another group of parasitic pathogens. Tapeworms and roundworms, the most commonly known helminths, can attack and colonize the intestinal tract, the liver, lungs, blood, skin layers, and brain. The immune system recognizes and responds to the presence of helminths as it does to other pathogens. But like bacteria and protozoa, certain helminths have evolved intricate mechanisms to protect themselves from attack by immune cells.

As many as 300 million people worldwide are believed to be infected by helminths known as blood flukes. One group of blood flukes called *schistosomes* invade the body by secreting a substance that softens skin tissue, allowing the parasites to enter. Once inside, schistosomes make their way through the bloodstream to the lungs and then on to the liver, where they mature into an adult form. The adult organisms take up permanent residence in the veins of the intestines draining the bladder. Adult schistosomes can live for many years in blood vessels that are filled with active phagocytes and other immune cells. What prevents these cells from destroying the invading schistosomes?

Researchers have discovered that schistosomes elude circulating immune cells by masquerading as host cells—cells that the body will recognize as "self." They accomplish this amazing feat by gathering substances shed from the surfaces of host cells and draping them around their outer membranes. When phagocytes or other immune cells come in contact with the disguised invaders, they can detect only self antigens and do not respond.

Before the schistosomes disguise themselves, however, the immune system will have had time to generate a response to the organism's original antigens. And although this initial response is not enough to destroy the invader, it does—in a fascinating way—allow both the host and the pathogen to survive. The immune system cannot destroy those resident schistosomes that have taken on a protective layer of host antigens. But the body can and does quickly respond to any new infection by undisguised schistosomes. Thus, while the infection remains chronic, it never reaches the stage where the life of the host is threatened. In this way, the disguised schistosomes, which cannot live in a dead host, insure their own survival.

The protozoa *Pneumocystis carinii* and *Toxoplasma gondii* are called *opportunists*—pathogens that cause disease only when the immune system of the host is compromised. For immunosuppressed or immunodeficient individuals, another group of opportunistic disease organisms, called *fungi,* pose a serious threat as well. Fungi are single-celled organisms, larger than bacteria. They exist all around us, in soil and water and vegetation, and even within us, on the skin and in the gastrointestinal tract.

Some fungi are potent enemies. During the Middle Ages, strange epidemics of a disease known today as *mycotoxicosis* swept through large parts of Europe. The disease began with a painful swelling of the hands, arms, feet, and legs. Gradually, as this swelling worsened, the pain—a terrible burning sensation—became agonizing. In the most severe cases, the affected tissues became dry and black and actually dropped from the body without any loss of blood. Pregnant women afflicted with the disease commonly suffered miscarriages. Other victims fell prey to wild, frightening convulsions. Over twenty outbreaks of this terrifying disease were recorded between 900 and 1254 A.D. The epidemic of 944 in Southern France is estimated to have killed 40,000 people. The disease came to be known as "St. Anthony's fire," because it was widely believed that the burning limbs were being consumed and reduced to charcoal by the Holy Fire. Sporadic outbreaks of St. Anthony's fire have continued even into this century, with the most recent in 1951.

The disease, we know today, is caused by a parasitic fungus, *Claviceps purpurea,* and is spread by the ingestion of contaminated grains. The fungus releases a group of substances called ergot alkaloids, which severely constrict blood vessels, causing the gangrene-like destruction of tissues. The ergot alkaloids also stimulate uterine contractions, causing spontaneous abortion in some cases. And recently we have discovered another curious fact: ergot alkaloids contain in their chemical structure lysergic acid—the major component of lysergic acid diethylamide, or LSD. The wild convulsions associated with St. Anthony's fire appear to be the effects of lysergic acid on the central nervous system.

Fortunately, St. Anthony's fire is the exception. Of more than 100,000 identifiable species of fungi (commonly known as yeast and molds), only about 100 are known to cause disease in humans or animals. And in most cases human fungal infections are mild, limited to the hair, nails, or superficial layers of the skin. Often referred to as ringworm infections, these superficial fungi can involve the toes and feet ("athlete's foot"), or the scalp, nails, or groin ("jock itch"). Because these fungi do not invade the body, they pose little problem in and of themselves.

Candida albicans, another fungus, commonly resides in small numbers in the mouth, gastrointestinal tract, and vagina. Properly functioning, the body's immune system keeps the growth of *Candida* under control. When the immune system is compromised, however, fungi can be life-threatening. Patients with suppressed immune responses, for example, are at risk of contracting several sometimes fatal fungal infections—including a form of *Candida* infection that spreads to the kidneys, causing fever, shock, and in some cases death. The fungus *Cryptococcus neoformans,* a yeast organism found in infected pigeon feces, can cause a deadly form of meningitis—an inflammation of the envelope that surrounds the brain and spinal cord. The fungus *Aspergillus* is commonly found in most healthy adults. But in immunosuppressed or immunodeficient patients, *Aspergillus* frequently causes a fungal infection of the lungs and other organs which can prove fatal.

The body's enemies are many. Disease-producing agents invade across wide-ranging borders, attacking and destroying in a variety of ways. The threat to the body is constant and ever-changing. Not only must we defend ourselves against pathogens that have plagued human life for eons, but also against invaders that are utterly new—mutated viral and bacterial strains, or industrial contaminants that the body has never before encountered in the hundreds of thousands of years of its evolution. The challenge of defense is enormous. To meet this challenge, the body has evolved a highly complex and dynamic arsenal of weapons and strategies—the human immune system.

three

THE ARSENAL OF DEFENSE

There is at bottom only one genuinely scientific treatment for all diseases and that is to stimulate the phagocytes.

GEORGE BERNARD SHAW
The Doctor's Dilemma

With the single exception of the intricate network of neurons that gives us the capacity to think, feel and speak, no other system in the body is so elaborately interconnected or so finely tuned as the human immune system.

Paradoxically, the immune system begins with relatively few basic components. The weapons in the body's arsenal of defense include a limited number of specialized cells, and substances produced by cells. *Phagocytes* possess the ability to engulf and destroy invading viruses, bacteria, fungi, protozoa, and helminths, as well as cellular debris that washes into the bloodstream. They are joined by *killer T cells* and *natural killer cells,* which are programmed to seek out and destroy virally invaded cells and cancer cells. And a third group, the *B cells*, may also join the battle by producing antibodies, specialized proteins which can neutralize and destroy, through a variety of strategies, a wide range of disease-producing microbes.

Out of these few components, the body has evolved two major strategies of defense against disease—*cellular immunity* and *humoral immunity.* Cellular immunity involves the recruitment of phagocytes, killer T cells, and natural killer cells. This form of immune response pits these immune cells against invading pathogens in direct combat. Vertebrates and invertebrates alike possess the mechanisms of cellular immunity, suggesting that it is the oldest form of defense against microbial attack. Cellular immunity may in fact have evolved from one of the earliest defense mechanisms, *inflammation.* In nonspecific inflammation, the body responds to cuts or abrasions by enlisting a variety of specialized cells to repair the damaged tissue; their activity is often visible in the familiar swelling and reddening of the skin. Specific inflammation, on the other hand, is more complex, involving not only these specialized inflammatory cells but also the cells of the immune system. Specific inflammation generates immunologic memory of the foreign cell or substance that triggered the response. Should that foreign cell or substance invade the body again, the specific inflammatory response will occur more rapidly and with greater force. In some disease states, specific inflammation can become chronic and destructive. But in most cases, both specific and nonspecific inflammation are potent strategies for defense.

With the evolution of vertebrate life, a second system of defense evolved, more powerful than cellular immunity: the production of antibodies, proteins designed to neutralize the invading organism. The strategy of antibody production, a kind of cellular chemical warfare, is called humoral immunity (the term derives from "humor," which refers to any functioning fluid in the body).

The Russian zoologist Elie Metchnikoff was the first to glimpse the mechanisms of cellular immunity, more than a hundred years ago. In 1882, he made a startling observation while studying the larvae of transparent starfish. Somewhat poetically placing a rose thorn into a larva, he found that specialized cells of the larva completely surrounded the thorn in a matter of hours —just the way a defense force might surround an enemy intruder. Curious, Metchnikoff injected various colored dyes into the starfish larvae. The result was the same: the larval cells surrounded and engulfed the dyes.

With growing interest, Metchnikoff extended his study to a small water flea called *Daphnia.* He introduced pathogenic fungal cells into the blood of this tiny animal and then watched as certain blood cells began to engulf and destroy the fungus. A nagging idea suddenly seemed more than a wild surmise: perhaps these blood cells actually protected the organism from disease by surrounding and destroying invading substances. Two years later, while experimenting with cells from rabbits as well as humans, Metchnikoff found the same mechanism at work: certain cells in the blood were able to engulf and destroy pathogenic bacteria. Metchnikoff discovered that this response was most evident in animals either recovering from an infection or recently injected with microorganisms. He gave the process the name *phagocytosis,* or "cell-eating." And he formulated a revolutionary theory: the body's main defense against bacterial infection, Metchnikoff argued, was based on the ability of phagocytes to engulf and destroy pathogenic organisms.

With the formulation of this theory, modern immunology was born.

Today we know that phagocytes are produced in the bone marrow and are present not only in the blood, but in all tissues of the body. Their activities represent one of the body's basic strategies for defense. Detecting an infection, nearby phagocytes migrate swiftly to the site of invasion. There, they will confront the enemy directly. Binding to a foreign cell, a phagocyte wraps its own cell membrane around the invader, trapping it inside. Chemical substances within the phagocyte then break down and destroy the components of the invading cell. A phagocyte literally eats the enemy, digesting and metabolizing its materials.

Bacteria, fungi, protozoa, and helminths are a phagocyte's prime targets. But phagocytes are nonspecific in their attack, consuming all types of pathogens, cellular debris, and even inert particles such as silica and asbestos. Pathogenic organisms and airborne contaminants are most likely to enter the body through the lungs, and it is in the lungs that phagocytes are most active. They swarm through the bronchial tissues, ceaselessly clearing and cleansing them. Lungs blackened with the particulate contaminants of cigarette smoke, for example, will slowly return to their normal pink color and spongy texture once the inhalation of smoke is stopped—thanks to the cleansing activities of phagocytes. Large numbers of phagocytes are also present in the liver. There, among a variety of tasks, they rid the blood of cellular debris picked up as it courses through the body's tissues.

Studying the activity of phagocytes, Metchnikoff recognized two distinct cell types—those he called *macrophages,* or "big eaters," and those he called *granulocytes* (cells that are now known as *neutrophils*). Under the microscope they appeared structurally quite distinct. But at work, both types of phagocytes seemed to do exactly the same thing: engulf and destroy foreign cells and substances. And for the better part of a century, researchers continued to assume that granulocytes and macrophages performed one role in immune responses: phagocytosis.

Over the last decade, however, exciting breakthroughs in immunology have forced researchers to look more closely at the lowly macrophage. We now know that these extraordinary cells play a far more embracing role in the entire spectrum of immune responses. Indeed, we have come to believe that macrophages—the first cells identified with the body's defense against disease—may well be the one *absolutely essential* component of the immune system. While certain animals survive without active T cell populations, and others survive without the help of antibody-producing B cells, no vertebrate on earth has ever been observed to exist without active macrophages.

The reason is a fundamental one. Macrophages initiate and enhance the activities of virtually every other cell of the immune system. Without the help of macrophages, for example, T cells would never recognize the antigen molecules that alert them to the presence of foreign substances or cells. And without T cell recognition, the production of antibodies by B cells would never commence. Indeed, the full range of immune responses depends on the activity of macrophages. And the entire cycle begins when macrophages at the site of an infection alert arriving T cells to the presence of an invader.

T lymphocytes, like all immune cells, are formed in the bone marrow. From there, immature T cells, called *prothymocytes,* migrate to the thymus, a small organ situated just above the heart. In the thymus, these immature and immunologically incompetent T cells develop into fully functional "helper," "killer," or "suppressor" T cells. Each of these three separate populations go on to play very distinct, though interacting, roles in immune responses.

But what all T cells have in common, and what sets them apart from phagocytes—indeed, what qualifies them as a central marvel of nature—is their ability to recognize the precise identity of an invading organism or foreign substance. They do so via a set of molecules carried on the surface of each T cell membrane. This set of molecules, called a *T cell receptor,* is genetically designed to recognize a single unique molecular combination. Like a precision lock, a T cell receptor can be turned by only one key: a specific antigen. This lock and key characteristic of T cell receptors and antigens carries a staggering implication. Scientists estimate that there are more than one million potential antigens, one million different kinds of molecules—from ragweed pollen to the surface antigens of microbes and virally infected cells—that will mark them as foreign, and to which the body will react by triggering an immune response. Because each T cell is specific for only one unique antigen, the immune system has evolved at least one million distinct subgroups of T cells—each subgroup genetically designed to recognize one of the one million potential antigens. Precisely how the body has evolved the ability to respond to so vast a range of enemies is not fully known.

Once helper T cells have matured in the thymus, they enter the bloodstream and lymph system, where they begin to circulate through the tissues of the body. Each helper T cell, through its receptor, is exquisitely alert to the presence of the single antigen it was designed to recognize. The vast number of these specialized cells and their progeny will circulate through the blood and tissues of the body for a lifetime, rarely encountering that single, unique antigen, rarely expressing their biological potential. But when a helper T cell does come in contact with the antigen specific for its receptor—when the helper T cell programmed to recognize a hepatitis B virus antigen encounters the hepatitis-infected cell, for example—that T cell awakens from a suspended state into vigorous life. Activated, the helper T cell begins to marshal the forces of other immune cells to battle.

For a time it was believed that the activation of helper T cells was simply a matter of their coming in contact with antigen molecules on an invading organism. But recent research has described a far more complicated process: the activation, in fact, requires a complex interaction among helper T cells, antigen, and macrophages. Macrophages are not themselves antigen-specific—that is, they do not possess the ability to recognize distinct foreign antigens. But they do possess the ability to concentrate antigens and present them to T cells. Without the help of macrophages at the site of infection, T cells simply would not respond to the antigens present and the complex cycle of T and B cells would never begin.

The interaction of macrophages and helper T cells illustrates one of many complex relationships among the cells of the immune system. As we have seen, helper T cells require the activity of macrophages in order to respond to antigens. And in much the same way, macrophages themselves require the presence of the very T cells they have activated in order to complete the job of engulfing and destroying certain pathogenic organisms. This can be seen most clearly in immunodeficient individuals whose macrophage populations may remain intact, but whose helper T cell functions are impaired. Without the assistance of helper T cells, macrophages may engulf certain pathogens, but they cannot destroy them. Indeed, the pathogens actually continue to grow within the macrophage cell. *Mycobacterium tuberculosis,* for example, possesses the ability to live and grow within macrophages in the lungs. By mechanisms we do not yet understand, these bacteria then induce macrophages to produce and release substances that contribute to the severe pulmonary inflammation of tuberculosis. A number of other pathogenic bacteria, fungi, and protozoa can exist within macrophages; their destruction requires the presence of activated helper T cells.

As their name implies, helper T cells do not participate directly in the attack and destruction of disease-producing organisms. Rather, like generals in the field, they issue the commands that initiate and direct the activities of other immune cells. At the site of an infection, activated helper T cells begin to reproduce. Some of these newly produced helper T cells will remain at the site of the infection, assisting macrophages in their counterattack. Other helper T cells will migrate through the bloodstream to the spleen and nearby lymph nodes. There they will trigger the production of the second major T cell population: specialized attack cells called killer T cells.

Like helper and suppressor T cells, the precursors of killer T cells mature in the thymus. They migrate to the lymph nodes and spleen, the major sites of immunologic activity when the immune system is confronted with a pathogenic virus. There, these precursor cells will reside, endowed with the biological potential for battle, but dormant until activated helper T cells arrive from the site of infection and make contact with them. Precursor T cells are already programmed for a specific antigen. An activated helper T cell specific for the hepatitis B virus antigen will activate only precursor killer T cells specific for the same antigen. Contact between the two antigen-specific cells triggers the final development of fully functional killer T cells, which then move out of the lymph nodes and spleen and speed toward the site of infection. Like helper T cells, killer T cells bear on their cell membranes antigen-specific receptors that allow them to detect the presence of a specific antigen on the surface of an invaded host cell. At the moment of recognition, killer T cells bind themselves to the surface of the invaded cells, setting in motion a series of chemical reactions that will lead inexorably to the destruction of that cell. These chemical reactions, mediated by the killer T cell, attack the membrane that surrounds the invaded cell, breaking through it and releasing the cell's essential components. Viruses spilling out of such cells are prey to attack by phagocytes and antibodies.

Killer T cells are the body's most potent weapon against viral infection and certain types of cancer cells. They are joined in the battle of cell against cell by a third type of immune cell, one whose nature still remains a provocative puzzle to researchers—the natural killer cell.

Immunologists first glimpsed the activity of these powerful cells in experiments with a strain of laboratory mice known as "beige" mice. These inbred mice are far more susceptible to developing viral infections and certain kinds of tumors than other strains of laboratory mice. Their heightened susceptibility mirrors the clinical condition of a human disease called

Chediak-Higashi syndrome, in which patients are susceptible to recurrent infections and a strikingly high incidence of cancer. When the disease syndromes were first recognized, immunologists were at a loss to explain the cause. Both beige mice and individuals with Chediak-Higashi syndrome have normal populations of T cells and B cells. Why, then, are they prey to certain viruses and tumors?

Immunologic studies soon revealed that Chediak-Higashi patients and beige mice have at least one common immunologic defect: they both lack a population of specialized immune cells that have come to be called natural killer cells.

Experiments with another strain of laboratory mice, called "nude" mice, have confirmed the importance of natural killer cells in the body's defense. Nude mice lack a thymus, the organ in which immature T cells develop into helper, killer, and suppressor T cells. And as a result, nude mice are without a mature T cell population. Yet even without these powerful cells, nude mice have no greater incidence of tumors than immunologically normal mice. The reason, we now know, is that nude mice are protected by the presence of active natural killer cells.

Immunologists understand very little about how natural killer cells recognize foreign cells and cancer cells. We do know that a single natural killer cell can target and destroy cancer cells as well as cells infected with different viruses; but how it recognizes these enemies and distinguishes them from the body's own cells remains a mystery. Obviously its methods are different from the lock and key specificity of T cell antigen recognition. Each natural killer cell can target a broad range of enemy cells—and that diversity gives it a crucial advantage. Unlike killer T cells, natural killer cells do not have to be activated by helper T cells in order to develop. They appear to be ready to respond at every moment to the presence of a tumor cell or virally infected cell. This "quick strike" capacity can be of critical importance against rapidly proliferating enemies. Many scientists have begun to suspect, in fact, that natural killer cells have the primary responsibility for immune surveillance against the rise of cancer cells in the body.

Natural killer cells, killer T cells, and phagocytes comprise the body's arsenal of cellular immunity. Elie Metchnikoff argued, more than a century ago, that cellular immunity represented the body's sole mechanism of defense against disease. But even as he was formulating his theories, other researchers were making new and startling observations that could not be explained by the mechanisms of cellular immunity.

In 1888, George Nuttall, an American bacteriologist working in Germany, made a provocative discovery. He found that when he removed serum (the fluid phase of blood) from animals that had survived a bacterial infection and then added the infecting bacteria to the serum, the bacteria were quickly destroyed—even though serum contained absolutely no immune cells. Six years later, Richard Pfeiffer and Vasily Isaeff confirmed that some unknown mechanism, one that did not involve the direct attack by immune cells, was at work in the body's defense. They observed that *Vibrio cholerae,* the cholera bacterium, could be destroyed simply by placing it in the serum taken from immunized guinea pigs. These studies also revealed that the unknown factor at work in the serum was exquisitely specific: it would kill only the bacteria used to infect the animal from which the immune serum was obtained. Something in that serum, something quite apart from the phagocytes Metchnikoff had first observed, was capable of destroying bacteria. Researchers in the last years of the nineteenth century termed this mysterious substance *antibody*. The activity of antibodies—the destruction of pathogens not by cells, but by a chemical substance—came to be called *humoral immunity*.

Bitter debates raged between the proponents of cellular immunity and humoral immunity—but not for long. For while proponents of one theory or the other zealously defended their own research, macrophages went on engulfing and destroying pathogenic organisms; and in the absence of immune cells, certain substances were observed to neutralize and destroy bacteria, fungi, and protozoa. The evidence of *both* cellular immunity and humoral immunity was incontrovertible.

The remarkable fact is that the body depends for its defense not on one strategy alone, but on two very distinct parallel strategies. Indeed, both kinds of immune responses often work together in the battle against a single infection. Antibodies can actually enhance the phagocytic activities of macrophages, for example. And the more we have learned in the last several decades about the complex interaction between the two strategies, the more we have come to realize how inextricably bound together are *all* the components of the immune system.

The principal agents of humoral immunity, as the early researchers recognized, are substances known as antibodies (or *immunoglobulins*, as they are also called). Antibodies are produced by a specialized group of lymphocyte cells called B cells. Generated in the bone marrow, B cells migrate directly to the spleen and to lymph nodes throughout the body, where they remain, awaiting the arrival of activated T cells. B cells, like all lymphocytes, are antigen-specific. A B cell programmed to produce antibodies against the hepatitis B virus antigen, for example, will be activated only by the presence of that single antigen. Helper T cells trigger the dormant B cells in much the same way they trigger killer T cells—simply by making contact across antigen receptor sites on their cell membranes. Activated by contact with arriving helper T cells, B cells direct their components and energy to one purpose—the production of antibodies.

Antibodies are complex protein molecules constructed, like all proteins, of amino acids. There are some twenty different amino acids, and the nature and shape of a protein is dictated by their sequence. Small proteins may be composed of fewer than thirty amino acids; larger proteins may combine more than five thousand. Proteins that share the same sequence of amino acids will assume the same form.

Antibody molecules are composed of four strands of amino acids which, twisted together, assume the shape of the letter Y. In an antibody molecule, form and function are very nearly one. The two arms of the antibody protein, like the claws of a lobster, make contact with the external environment. Small pockets along these arms, made up of the twists and folds of strings of amino acids, can bind with antigens. Each unique antibody can bind only one specific antigen molecule. The overwhelming number of contacts the antibody will make are with substances that do not fit precisely into its antigen-binding site. In these blind collisions, the molecules merely glance off one another and go on their way, unaltered. When an antibody encounters the antigen for which it is specific, however, the two molecules will bind together; and at that moment any of a number of different destructive strategies may be set in motion.

When antibodies bind to the surface antigens of bacteria,

fungi, or protozoa, they firmly anchor the pathogen so that phagocytes can more easily engulf and destroy the invaders. Circulating antibodies, binding with viral antigens, can prevent the virus from binding to the body's cells. And in the battle against toxin-producing bacteria, antibodies can actually bind to the toxins themselves, neutralizing them and preventing them from reaching sensitive tissues and cells.

But circulating antibodies can also participate in the direct attack and destruction of invading pathogens. Their strategy is unlike any other in the body's immunologic arsenal. Binding to the surface of a target cell, an antibody molecule triggers a complex chemical reaction that will, at its conclusion, literally blast the enemy cell apart. The explosive ingredient in this reaction is a distinct class of circulating proteins, called *complement proteins,* produced by both macrophages and liver cells.

There are at least fifteen different kinds of complement proteins. On their own, circulating through the bloodstream, individual complement molecules are inert, inactive. They might seem, at first glance, to have no purpose at all—that is, until an antibody molecule binds to an invading cell. The binding of antibody with antigen triggers a chemical reaction that attracts the complement protein called C1, drawing it out of circulation and inducing it to make contact with the antibody molecule on the cell membrane of the invader. The joining of C1 then attracts a cascading sequence of more complement proteins—C2, C3, and C4—ready to bind to the new aggregate of antibody and C1 attached to the cell membrane. As C2 and C4 complement proteins arrive, C1, like a skilled surgeon, cuts each of the molecules into two pieces. One half floats off in the bloodstream; the others, joining with C1, form a growing aggregate on the surface of the target cell, which then attracts C3 out of circulation. Part of the C3 molecule floats away; part of it, like the others, binds, creating a new aggregate that attracts and binds C5. The cascading sequence continues as more complement proteins—C6, C7, and C8—are attracted to the cell.

In this complex sequence, each complement protein *must* be activated in the right order, and under the right circumstances, for the complement reaction to proceed. Strictly speaking, the binding of complement is not a single event but a dynamic process—a cascading sequence which, for all its complexity, occurs in less than a second, long before the invading cell has a chance to escape. Each arriving complement protein alters the nature of the growing aggregate, eventually transforming it into a small explosive device. With the arrival and binding of the last complement protein, C9, a chemical reaction detonates the aggregate, blasting a small but lethal hole through the membrane of the invading cell. This process, repeated thousands of times across the surface of the cell, bursts the cell membrane, releasing the contents of the cell into the environment.

The site of an infection or inflammation is littered with active and inactive pieces of complement; and curiously, the very presence of individual complement proteins can help bring on the destruction of invading microbes. Complement molecules possess a unique affinity for almost any foreign surface. Bound to the surface of a bacterial cell, for example, pieces of complement seem to attract nearby phagocytes, drawing them to the invader and enhancing their ability to engulf and destroy.

From the binding of complement proteins to the ability to attract phagocytes to pathogenic cells, antibody molecules perform a variety of defense functions. Based on their specific function and structural differences, antibodies are classified into five distinct groups. When an individual is first exposed to a particular antigen, for example, B cells begin to produce a class of antibodies called immunoglobulin M, or IgM. IgM antibodies are extremely efficient in triggering the complement system: a single IgM molecule, binding itself to a surface antigen, can initiate the entire complement cascade. As immune responses proceed, or during a second exposure to the same antigen, B cells begin to produce a second class of antibodies, called immunoglobulin G. IgG antibodies account for about three-quarters of the antibodies present in the bloodstream. Like IgM, IgG is important in initiating the complement cascade. But IgG has a unique property. Because of its special structure, it is the only class of antibody that can cross the placenta. Thus, IgG is responsible for protecting the fetus as well as the newborn infant from infection while their own immune systems are developing. A third class of antibodies, immunoglobulin A, is found predominantly in body secretions such as saliva, tears, and nasal fluids. IgA antibodies represent the first line of defense against infection. Secreted along mucous membranes, IgA antibodies have the ability to neutralize invading viruses before they can enter the body. Immunoglobulin D, a fourth class of antibodies, appears structurally distinct from the others, although its functions in immune responses have not yet been identified. The final class of antibodies, immunoglobulin E, is known to be important in triggering allergic reactions.

During its life, a single B cell is capable of producing antibody molecules from several immunoglobulin classes. In an immune response against the hepatitis B virus, for example,

IgM and IgG antibodies may be produced sequentially by a single B cell, both targeted to the hepatitis B antigen. When first activated, a B cell will produce IgM antibodies. Antibody production will switch to IgG as the immune response gathers strength, progressing on through a sequence of antibody classes dictated by the particular defense strategy of the immune response. Curiously, once a B cell has switched from the production of IgM to IgG, it cannot go back to producing IgM. For unknown reasons, B cell production of antibodies can only go forward through the sequence of immunoglobulin classes.

Set in motion, the body's arsenal of defense—phagocytes, killer T cells, natural killer cells, and antibodies—is enormously powerful. And its power comes, in part, from its exquisite flexibility in responding to infection. Virtually every cell of the immune system has the power to assist and enhance the activities of every other cell. In the intricate dynamics of a gathering immune response, one cell will activate another, which then activates a third, which may in turn enhance or assist the first. Working in concert, the cells of the immune system are capable of enormous violence. The combined forces of the immune system can be so powerful and destructive, in fact, that a separate and distinct contingent of immune cells exists for the sole purpose of controlling immune responses—literally "turning off" the activities of helper T cells and antibody-producing B cells when the job of defense is accomplished. These cells, called suppressor T cells, are one of the three populations of T cells that leave the thymus at maturity. Without them, the massive power of an immune response, building on itself, would spiral out of control, turning the attack on an invader into an attack on the body itself.

Suppressor T cells have the ability to prevent helper T cells from triggering killer T cells and B cells in the lymph nodes. By releasing certain regulatory substances, suppressor T cells can also slow or stop B cell production of antibodies. Their power is enormous. They can bring to a halt the entire range of immune responses against an infection. Indeed, suppressor T cells are so powerful that the immune system has devised an intricate feedback system by which certain suppressor T cells monitor the effects of other suppressor T cells. If these cells begin to shut down an immune response too early, the monitoring cells will inhibit the activity of the suppressor T cells themselves.

The complex interaction of helper T cells and suppressor T cells, the "on" and "off" switch of immune responses, establishes one of the delicate and critical balances of the immune system. In healthy individuals, there are usually between two and three times as many helper T cells as suppressor T cells. That ratio may vary. In the aftermath of an infection, for example, a larger proportion of suppressor T cells may be present. When the ratio of helper and suppressor T cells is chronically upset, however—as it is among patients with Acquired Immune Deficiency Syndrome—the immune system itself can be seriously compromised. In some cases, AIDS patients exhibit reversed T cell counts: two to three times as many suppressor T cells as helper T cells. And in the last stages of the disease, AIDS patients may be virtually without detectable helper T cells. Immune responses are then continuously and severely suppressed, and AIDS patients become prey to a wide range of viral, fungal, bacterial, and protozoal infections.

Immunologists do not yet understand precisely how suppressor T cells know when to shut down an immune response, or how they exert their control over other cells. The solutions to some of these mysteries may shed new light on the mystery of how cancer cells manage to evade the immunologic defense system. As we have seen, killer T cells and natural killer cells can target, attack, and destroy tumor cells in the body. And yet in certain cases, for reasons we do not understand, tumor cells are able to evade the attack of these immune cells. Current research points toward a provocative possibility: suppressor T cells may actually work too well in certain circumstances, undermining the body's surveillance against tumor cells by suppressing the generation of killer T cells. We know, for example, that mice with active tumors have suppressor T cells in their spleens that specifically block the ability of the immune system to attack and kill the tumor cells. Scientists have actually been able to retard the growth of tumors by surgically removing the spleens, and with them large populations of suppressor T cells, from these animals. There is even evidence that the tumor cells themselves may be able to increase the number of suppressor T cells—evading the immune system by turning its arsenal against the body itself.

The strength and success of an immune response depends on the recruitment of large numbers of immune cells. Once immune responses have successfully defended the body against infection, and suppressor T cells have slowed the activity of immune cells, most of the cells generated for the immune response begin to die off, no longer necessary to fight an immediate threat. But a special contingent of T and B cells remains—cells that will protect the body if the same invading organism attacks again.

These cells are no different from the other helper and killer

T cells and B cells that were produced to fight the invader. They each possess receptor sites genetically programmed to recognize the unique antigens of the pathogen. But there is one crucial difference: these *memory cells,* instead of dying off, will continue to live for long periods in the body. After an acute infection has been beaten back by the immune system, large numbers of the same T and B cells that were generated to fight the original infection will remain in the bloodstream and lymph system. Before the first infection, there may have been one helper T cell in one million programmed to recognize the antigen of the hepatitis B virus; after the infection there will be thousands more of these antigen-specific cells. Should the invading organism return, they will be instantly mobilized to mount a far more rapid and efficient counterattack. Memory T cells will immediately activate macrophages and B cells. Memory B cells will start the production of antibody against the invader. In the battle against rapidly proliferating viruses or a highly toxic bacteria, the advantage of a defense force of memory cells can be critical.

The activity of memory cells is illustrated dramatically in an immune reaction called the *Koch phenomenon,* which serves as the basis for the familiar tuberculin skin test for tuberculosis. Robert Koch, one of the pioneers of immunology, first identified the bacterium responsible for tuberculosis in 1882. In early experiments, he injected laboratory guinea pigs with the bacteria and observed that a small nodule formed at the site of the injection within about ten to fourteen days. Within six to twelve weeks the infection had spread to the animals' lymph nodes, and before long, all of the animals were dead. Koch repeated the experiment, injecting a second group of animals with tuberculosis; but this time, several weeks after the first injection, he inoculated the same animals again at a different site. And he observed a curious phenomenon. As in the first inoculation, a nodule appeared at the second injection site. But this time, the nodule appeared very quickly—within one or two days. And unlike the first nodule, the second soon healed. The body had apparently walled off this second inoculation and prevented the further spread of the pathogen.

Koch guessed correctly that the localized skin reaction he had observed was some sort of immune response; but the exact mechanism remained a mystery to him. Today, we know that the Koch phenomenon depends upon the presence of already activated T cells. The first injection of tuberculosis in Koch's laboratory animals triggered their immune systems. But the job of mounting a defense took time. More than a week passed before inflammation appeared at the site of infection—evidence of the activity of immune cells—but by then the bacteria had been able to infect the lymph nodes. When Koch administered the second inoculation, however, large numbers of activated T cells were already present in the bloodstream. Moving swiftly and in great numbers, these memory cells were able to wall off the second infection within one or two days.

A similar process takes place in the tuberculin skin test. To perform the test, a physician injects a small amount of tuberculin, the inactivated tuberculosis antigen, under the skin. If the color and texture of the skin is unchanged after 24 to 48 hours, the test is negative; the immune system has not responded to the antigen, indicating that the individual has never been exposed to tuberculosis. If the site of the injection has become reddened, thickened, and hard to the touch, however, the test is positive. A positive response indicates that the body has reacted swiftly to the antigen, signaling a previous exposure to tuberculin. As a result of that previous exposure, memory cells were produced. With the injection of tuberculin, and a second exposure to the same antigen, these memory cells explode into action. The job of recruiting and stimulating nearby cells may take memory T cells anywhere from 12 to 24 hours. Inflammation caused by the newly recruited macrophages will usually reach its peak within another 24-hour period. As Koch observed, the sum of both responses requires between 24 and 48 hours.

The Koch phenomenon is an example of *delayed-type hypersensitivity,* a form of cellular immunity that occurs when any antigen is injected under the skin after a previous exposure. Physicians use similar tests—injecting common antigens of *Candida* or various *Streptococci,* to which virtually all individuals have been exposed, and then observing the body's reaction —as a measure of the strength of an individual's immune responses.

In an important sense, the immune system is far greater than the sum of its parts. For unlike the body's other major components (the respiratory system or digestive tract, for example), the immune system does not reside in a single organ or group of organs. From their genesis in the bone marrow, immune cells flow out into virtually every part of the body. The precursors of killer T cells and B cells move out into lymph nodes, where they will reside until they are called on to fight an infection. Other cells—phagocytes, helper T cells, and natural killer cells—circulate ceaselessly through the extended network of blood and lymph vessels.

No single organ controls and regulates immune responses. In a battle against the agents of disease, it is the immune cells themselves, responding moment by moment to the ever-changing threat, that regulate immune responses. Through a complex communications network of commands and counter-commands, carried out in a language of chemical reactions, immune cells shape the body's strategy against invasion even as the battle is being waged.

A century of observation and accumulating knowledge about the functioning of immune responses have provided immunologists with a good understanding of *what* the different cells of the immune system do to protect us against disease. But the fundamental question of *how* these cells work has remained, until very recently, unanswered. How, for example, do macrophages know to migrate toward a site of infection? And once they reach the infection, how do they alert circulating helper T cells to the presence of antigens? How do helper T cells, rushing from the site of an infection to the nearest lymph nodes, tell B cells to begin the production of antibody? And how do suppressor T cells turn off that same B cell antibody production once the enemy has been defeated? For almost as long as immunology has been a science, researchers simply have not known.

four

THE LANGUAGE OF IMMUNE RESPONSE

What is your substance where of you are made
That millions of strange shadows on you tend?

WILLIAM SHAKESPEARE

In 1932, two American researchers stumbled upon a discovery that would ultimately lead immunologists to an understanding of the fundamental processes that link immune cells and regulate immune responses. A. R. Rich and M. R. Lewis, like many researchers, were intrigued by the Koch phenomenon—the localized skin response that followed a second exposure to tuberculin. They wanted to learn exactly *how* tuberculin produced the reddening and swelling recognized as delayed-type hypersensitivity.

The two researchers began their experiments by removing spleens from a small group of laboratory guinea pigs and cutting the organs into small fragments. Spleens were chosen because, like the lymph nodes, they serve as a storehouse for immune cells in the body. For investigators, the spleen provides a rich and easily isolated source of macrophages and T cells. Rich and Lewis placed the spleen fragments in glass dishes and covered them with a sterile broth. Over the next twenty-four hours, the researchers observed an intriguing reaction. Individual immune cells, both macrophages and T cells, began to migrate slowly out of the spleen fragments and across the surface of the dishes. Rich and Lewis then repeated the experiment using spleen fragments from guinea pigs that had been inoculated previously with tuberculin. Once again these sensitized T cells and macrophages moved out of the spleens and across the surface of the dishes.

The migration of the immune cells was an unexpected observation. But what Rich and Lewis discovered next was truly provocative. Again they isolated spleen fragments from animals inoculated with tuberculin, but this time they added tuberculin to the culture dish as well. In effect, Rich and Lewis duplicated Koch's second inoculation, not in laboratory animals, but in a culture of immune cells. To their great surprise, the investigators now observed that only the T cells migrated out of the spleen fragments and across the dishes. The macrophages stayed exactly where they were, immobilized in the spleen fragments. Rich and Lewis repeated their experiment, always with the same results. In the absence of tuberculin, sensitized macrophages and T cells alike moved slowly across the culture dish. But when tuberculin was added to the culture, only the T cells migrated. The macrophages remained immobilized. Why? What inhibited the movement of macrophages in the presence of tuberculin?

Rich and Lewis had no answers. Tuberculin obviously had

a dramatic effect on certain cells of the immune system. The researchers were convinced that what they had seen in the culture dishes related in some way to the skin response that Koch had observed when he injected tuberculin under the skin of laboratory animals. But the larger picture of the underlying immune responses involved seemed confusing. In the Koch phenomenon, a tuberculin inoculation appeared to *attract* immune cells to the site of the injection, which then became inflamed. But in Rich and Lewis's laboratory dish, tuberculin appeared to *inhibit* the movement of at least one kind of immune cell, the macrophage.

For more than two decades, questions raised by the Rich and Lewis study challenged immunologists. Then in 1966, two research groups, working independently, began to piece together a solution. They started simply by repeating the original experiments, with variations made possible by new laboratory techniques. Instead of using fragments of spleens, the scientists prepared solutions containing large numbers of T cells and macrophages in suspension. They placed portions of these cell suspensions inside small glass capillary tubes (tubes that resemble slender glass straws). These tubes were then placed in the bottom of laboratory dishes containing a sterile broth. By using the capillary tubes, investigators could measure more accurately the actual distance over which the immune cells migrated.

Initial results confirmed the Rich and Lewis findings. When the investigators placed in suspension immune cells from naive animals—animals that had never been exposed to tuberculin—both macrophages and T cells began to migrate across the surface of the culture dishes. When tuberculin was added to the same cultures of naive immune cells, the immune cells also migrated. But when tuberculin was added to cells from animals previously inoculated with tuberculin, only the T cells migrated. The macrophages remained immobilized in the capillary tubes.

To insure that these effects were not specific to tuberculin itself, the investigators repeated their experiments using other antigens. The results were always the same. All that was required was that the laboratory animals be exposed to the antigen beforehand. Then, when immune cells were removed and placed in a culture with that antigen, macrophages were blocked from migrating. It seemed clear that some form of immunity must be triggering the reaction. And the investigators guessed that the process involved memory T cells sensitized by the first exposure to the antigen.

They then made a discovery that would begin a revolution in immunology. Once again the researchers isolated T cells and macrophages from previously inoculated animals and placed these cells in dishes that contained nutrient broth and tuberculin. Instead of measuring immune cell migration, however, they simply separated out the culture broth after about twenty-four hours. This broth contained no cells at all—only the original nutrients, tuberculin, and any substances that might have been secreted by the T cells and macrophages. The broth was then added to culture dishes containing immune cells from naive animals. These cells had no immunologic memory of tuberculin—no memory cells that specifically recognized the tuberculin antigen. Given the results of previous experiments, the broth should have no inhibitory effect at all.

But when the culture broth was added to the naive immune cells, and the laboratory dishes were placed under the microscope, the investigators were astonished by what they saw. The T cells had migrated outward, just as before. But the macrophages remained completely immobilized, inhibited from migrating out of the capillary tubes.

What most astonished the investigators was simply this: the macrophages that were blocked from migrating had come from animals *not* previously exposed to tuberculin. In all the earlier experiments, as far back as the Rich and Lewis studies, researchers had consistently found that macrophages from naive animals would migrate freely across the surface of the dishes, with or without the presence of an antigen. Now, to their surprise, they had discovered that something in the nutrient broth, presumably secreted either by macrophages or T cells, could actually inhibit the migration of macrophages that were not sensitized to tuberculin.

There seemed only one explanation for the new findings. The tuberculin in the first set of dishes must have stimulated the sensitized cells to release a substance, unrelated to a specific antigen, which, when it was added to the naive cells in the second set of dishes, inhibited the movement of macrophages. Using new techniques that enabled them to separate macrophages, T cells, and B cells, the investigators determined that this newly observed substance was produced by T cells. At the time, investigators knew nothing about its chemical makeup. All that was known was its extraordinary effect on macrophages. They called the new substance *migration inhibitory factor,* or MIF.

With the identification of migration inhibitory factor, questions that had baffled researchers for half a century began to find answers. It suddenly became clear why macrophages remain at the site of a delayed-type hypersensitivity reaction. T cells, activated by contact with an antigen, begin to secrete MIF; macrophages, passing through the site of infection, encounter this inhibitory substance and are quickly immobilized. In effect, migration inhibitory factor issues a command to arriving macrophages to stay and participate in the gathering immune response. Rich and Lewis had observed the inhibitory effect only in cells previously sensitized to tuberculin simply because large numbers of memory T cells in these cultures, already programmed to recognized tuberculin, had amplified the effect. But it was clear that any T cell, activated by an antigen, would release MIF.

The discovery of migration inhibitory factor ushered in a new era in immunology. Scientists had at last broken the code by which immune cells communicate with each other. The first "word" in the language of immune responses had been deciphered, a chemical command passed from T cell to macrophage. Even more important, immunologists finally understood the nature of the words themselves: proteins secreted by immune cells. Because the first of these proteins to be identified, migration inhibitory factor, controlled the movement *(kinesis)* of lymphocytes, researchers called the substances *lymphokines.*

With profound excitement, researchers set about to discover what other words might exist in the vocabulary of the immune system.

A virtual explosion of discoveries took place in the next few years, as researchers throughout the world began to test nutrient broths derived from immune cell cultures to see what they might contain. T cells had been found to produce a lymphokine; now researchers wondered if the macrophage, already known to be an important participant in a variety of immune functions, might also produce a lymphokine. In 1972, two researchers at Yale University Medical School, Igal Gery and Byron Waksman, conducted an experiment based on the method that was quickly becoming standard procedure in lymphokine research. First, they isolated macrophages from laboratory animals and placed the cells in culture dishes that contained a nutrient broth. Later, they removed the broth. It was already well known that the presence of macrophages stimulated T cells to grow; Gery and Waksman wanted to test whether a macrophage-produced lymphokine was responsible. They added the nutrient broth taken from the macrophage culture to a culture of T cells removed from the thymus of laboratory mice. Normally, these immature T cells cease dividing and die within seventy-two hours after they are removed from the thymus. If macrophages did indeed produce a substance which stimulated the growth of T cells, then the addition of the macrophage culture broth would presumably enable the cells to survive longer.

After seventy-two hours, the T cells were still alive. Not only were they alive, they had increased in number as well. Obviously something in the macrophage culture broth, a unique lymphokine, had stimulated the growth of the T cells. Gery and Waksman called the new lymphokine *lymphocyte activating factor* (or LAF, as it was affectionately called by some investigators).

With the discovery of lymphocyte activating factor, researchers had found a second link between macrophages and T cells. It was now clear that these immune cells could engage in two-way communication. T cells arriving at a site of infection or inflammation release migration inhibitory factor, which issues the command for circulating macrophages to stay put and perform their immune functions. Macrophages drawn to the site of the infection release lymphocyte activating factor, stimulating T cells to grow. The growing number of T cells in turn produce more migration inhibitory factor, recruiting additional phagocytic macrophages to the site of an immune response and increasing the amounts of lymphocyte activating factor produced. In this way, the lymphokine cycle amplifies itself, strengthening the body's defensive response to an invader.

While Gery and Waksman conducted their experiments on LAF, other investigators were studying the role macrophages played in other aspects of immune response. And they began to report that the macrophage culture broth apparently contained additional factors that stimulated other types of immune responses. Very quickly, the list of lymphokines was growing longer and becoming more confusing. One factor was discovered which appeared to enhance the production of killer T cells. Another apparently stimulated B cells to grow and mature. Still another enhanced antibody synthesis. During this period, lymphokines were identified simply on the basis of their effect on immune cells. (Only later, as immunologists perfected biochemical techniques, were they able to study the nature of the protein molecules themselves and hence characterize the chemical structure of various lymphokines.) So the newly discovered factors produced by macrophages were given functional names like B cell activating factor, helper peak 1, T cell replacing factor III, and B cell differentiation factor. At scientific meetings, immunologists found themselves discussing a bewildering number of acronyms: LAF, BAF, TRF, BDF, MP, and HP-1.

At the same time, investigators studying the role of T cells in immune responses were discovering an equally large and baffling number of lymphokines apparently produced by T cells. In 1975, two independent research groups reported that T cells, like macrophages, appeared to secrete a lymphokine that stimulated T cells to grow. This new lymphokine was called thymocyte stimulating factor, or TSF. And within the next few years, other investigators identified additional lymphokines produced by T cells—among them substances that were dubbed T cell growth factor, co-stimulator, T cell mitogenic factor, and secondary cytotoxic T cell inducing factor—all of which seemed to have the same function: the stimulation of T cells.

In a few short years, lymphokine research had become extraordinarily complicated, and increasingly puzzling. Investigators began to wonder how a macrophage could produce so many different lymphokines. And they puzzled over why both T cells and macrophages would produce substances which performed essentially the same function—the stimulation of T cell growth, for example—in a duplication of effort that seemed wasteful and unnecessary. The identification of so many lymphokines, each with its own name and acronym, had created an immunologic Tower of Babel: investigators were increasingly confounded by so many substances. And lymphokine research, which had begun with such promise and excitement, was in danger of becoming mired in confusion.

The reasons for confusion were several. Immune cells can produce lymphokines only in extremely small amounts. In a 24-hour period, one *million* T cells or macrophages will produce at most only a few *hundredths* of *one-billionth* of an ounce (0.00000000002 oz.) of a particular lymphokine. The task of purifying sufficient quantities of these substances for chemical analysis requires extraordinarily sophisticated techniques. While a few investigators trained in biochemistry attempted the purification of particular lymphokines, they found it extremely difficult to prevent the loss of precious amounts of the substance at each step of the process. In the end, the investigators were usually left with very little lymphokine—and a great deal of frustration.

Lymphokine studies were also hampered by the extent to which immunology had become a highly specialized field. The new research on lymphokines suddenly demanded skills that most immunologists had not yet developed. Investigators well versed in the theories of immunology, for example, lacked the highly specialized training required to conduct the biochemical purification of lymphokines.

The fundamental character of modern scientific research contributed to the state of confusion as well. Many researchers had established their professional reputations by defining, characterizing and, of course, naming their own newly discovered lymphokines. Grant proposals had been accepted and research funds awarded to carry out the work of investigating *different* lymphocyte and macrophage substances. Researchers who had added a distinct name and acronym to the long list of supposed lymphokines necessarily argued for the importance of their particular factor in the overall range of immune responses. In effect, the professional interests of lymphokine researchers tended to proliferate and maintain the confounding number of individual lymphokines that had been identified.

Still, by 1979, progress in the biochemical analysis of lymphokines had reached a point at which it became evident that the circumscribed activities of T cells and macrophages simply could not possibly be associated with so many different protein products. By 1979, more than a hundred lymphokine names had been coined by various research groups. And as the characteristics of these different lymphokines were established, researchers found it more and more difficult to differentiate one supposed lymphokine from another. The stage was set for a new synthesis of data and ideas.

On May 27, 1979, immunologists from laboratories around the world gathered for the Second International Lymphokine Workshop in Ermatingen, Switzerland. The speakers reviewed the latest results from studies that spanned the full range of lymphokine research, often describing new experiments and presenting as yet unpublished findings. As they listened to the presentations and the discussion of one lymphokine after another, several of the researchers in attendance began to sort through the confusion of so many names and so many acronyms. They realized that a large number of lymphokines had been identified that were produced by macrophages and that stimulated T cells to grow. Another group of lymphokines, produced by T cells, appeared to have the same function. Could fifteen separate lymphokines be required to serve one purpose?

After the session, a group of seven investigators adjourned to a small pub next to the meeting hall and discussed a revolutionary idea: perhaps the "alphabet soup" of different T cell–stimulating factors that had evolved over the previous decade of research was in fact no more than many different names for a small number of distinct lymphokines. As these scientists reviewed the recent research, they became more convinced that there were in fact only two T cell–stimulating lymphokines, one secreted by macrophages, the other by T cells themselves. And they suggested that some sort of common pathway linked the two lymphokines, creating a reaction that began with the macrophage and ended with the T cell.

The idea was nothing more than a hypothesis, a synthesis of current research. But the seven investigators were so sure of its validity that they decided on the spot to give the two lymphokines new names—names that would not be associated with the "alphabet soup" of other lymphokine names. One of the scientists, Verner Paetkau, suggested the name "interleukin," because both of the lymphokines appeared to act as signals between ("inter") immune cells, or leucocytes ("leukin"). The lymphokine produced by macrophages was called *interleukin 1.* The lymphokine produced by T cells was called *interleukin 2.*

Time and a burst of new research were to prove the interleukin concept correct. After the Ermatingen workshop, many investigators participated in an exchange of highly purified lymphokine preparations. The preparations were tested and cross-tested in different types of immune responses, and the results were convincing: one researcher's LAF was indeed another's BAF or HP-1. The study provided sufficient data to transform the interleukin concept from a visionary guess into an established theory.

And before long, researchers pieced together the precise details of the relationship between interleukin 1 and interleukin 2. They found that interleukin 1, produced by macrophages, triggers T cells to produce interleukin 2; interleukin 2 then stimulates the T cells to grow. Without interleukin 1, T cells would be unable to produce interleukin 2. And without interleukin 2, these T cells would be unable to grow and fulfill their immunologic function.

With a growing sense of excitement, immunologists were assembling the picture of an intricate sequence of commands and countercommands that controls the strategies of the body's defense. T cells, making contact with a pathogenic organism, release migration inhibitory factor, which issues a command to arriving macrophages to stay and participate in the immune or inflammatory response. Macrophages in turn release interleukin 1, which triggers T cells at the site of infection to release interleukin 2, stimulating the growth of more T cells. Increased numbers of T cells are now available to stimulate killer T cells and trigger B cells to reproduce and manufacture antibodies. The growing population of T cells also releases additional quantities of migration inhibitory factor, recruiting new phagocytic macrophages. And the swelling ranks of macrophages will release increased amounts of interleukin 1, renewing and amplifying the complex chain reaction of lymphokine responses. Researchers were at last deciphering the fundamental language by which the components of the human immune system communicate across a vast cellular network—a network that, even greatly simplified, seemed breathtakingly complex.

As research continued, aided by new techniques that enabled immunologists to purify lymphokines in larger quantities for study, these simple protein substances revealed even more of their astonishing powers. The results of several recent studies, for example, have demonstrated a fascinating link between lymphokines and the brain—specifically, the region of the brain that controls body temperature and the development of fever.

Fever is commonly associated with infections of all types. But for many years investigators never clearly understood the relationship between infection and the development of fever. What causes the body to run a fever? And does the elevation of body temperature serve a useful purpose in the fight against infection?

In 1948, P. B. Beeson first discovered the existence of a substance that appeared to cause fever. When he extracted the substance from immune cells and injected it into a laboratory animal, he consistently observed an elevation in the animal's body temperature. Researchers later discovered that this fever-producing molecule, called the *endogenous pyrogen,* is produced by macrophages. But even more interesting was the discovery that endotoxins, one form of toxin produced by certain bacteria, appeared to stimulate production of this endogenous pyrogen.

For the first time, a clear-cut relationship was established between an infectious agent and fever. When certain types of bacteria invade the body, they shed endotoxins from their cell walls. Then, as macrophages make their way to the site of the bacterial infection, they come in contact with these endotoxins and are stimulated to produce the endogenous pyrogen. Molecules of endogenous pyrogen then enter the bloodstream, where they flow toward the brain. There, the fever-producing molecules activate the temperature control center, increasing body temperature. We now know that not only endotoxin-bearing bacteria, but a wide range of different pathogens appear to trigger macrophages to produce the endogenous pyrogen.

Following these discoveries, investigators set about to characterize the endogenous pyrogen molecule. Like the lymphokines interleukin 1 and interleukin 2, the endogenous pyrogen was a relatively small protein. Indeed, the fever-producing molecule was in many ways startlingly similar to interleukin 1. In 1979 and 1980, investigators at several laboratories independently ventured a guess that the endogenous pyrogen might in fact be the T cell activating lymphokine, interleukin 1. Subsequent research has confirmed that guess. The endogenous pyrogen is indeed interleukin 1.

But one important question remained. Why did the immune system contain a mechanism for raising body temperature? What function did fever itself serve?

During this period, other researchers were tackling a related question that would ultimately provide an answer. Investigating the relationship between temperature and lymphocyte activity, they discovered that these cells work better at slightly elevated temperatures. Phagocytes appear to engulf and destroy pathogens more efficiently; both T and B cells appear to grow faster when the body's temperature is raised. With that discovery, the long-standing puzzle of fever was solved. Macrophages, recognizing the presence of pathogens, release interleukin 1 to induce fever, which, as long as the fever remains slight and short-term, provides the optimal conditions for immune cells to attack and destroy the invaders.

More recently, researchers have discovered another way macrophages appear to help the body in its fight against disease. Muscular ache and weakness, like fever, are symptoms often associated with an infection, but the cause of the discomfort that most illness brings has remained unclear. New experiments demonstrate that interleukin 1, released into muscle tissue, can induce the breakdown of muscle protein. The ache and muscular weakness associated with infections appear to be the direct result of this breakdown, induced by the release of interleukin 1. Researchers suspect that the unpleasant symptoms of an illness may be part of a crucial defense tactic. The body needs a great deal of energy to fight infection. By breaking down muscle protein, interleukin 1 mobilizes the raw material to produce energy and the components necessary to mount an effective defense.

Lymphokines serve as the communication network between phagocytes, lymphocytes, and natural killer cells, as well as between the immune system and other parts of the body, as research into the nature of fever has demonstrated. But lymphokines do more than direct and control the strategies of immune cells. Immunologists have recently discovered a special group of lymphokines which themselves possess the extraordinary ability to attack and destroy cancer cells.

The trail that led to the discovery of these potent antitumor lymphokines has spanned two centuries. As far back as the 1700s, physicians were aware of an intriguing relationship between cancer and infectious disease. In a number of dramatic cases, when patients with certain kinds of tumors went on to develop serious bacterial infections, their tumors underwent complete remission. No one could explain the cause—but in 1891 a New York physician named William B. Coley decided to use the phenomenon as a treatment for cancer. One of Coley's patients had already undergone four operations, none of which had succeeded in slowing the growth of his tumors. Frustrated by failure, Coley took a gamble. He intentionally infected the patient with a species of bacteria known to cause remission in cancer patients. The gamble paid off. After resisting all attempts at surgery, the tumor regressed and disappeared, and the patient lived without any recurrence of the disease.

Coley had discovered an incredibly powerful weapon against cancer, but it was a weapon that would prove to be very difficult to control. In some patients, the technique brought about a remission of cancer; in other cases, the patients died from severe bacterial infections before the tumor itself was affected. Coley and other physicians soon discovered that they did not have to use living bacteria to achieve tumor remission. The broth removed from a culture of bacteria also had the power to destroy tumors, although these culture broths varied widely in both their potency and their effect on cancer cells. Nevertheless, Coley reported a significant number of well-documented successes using bacterial culture broths against tumors. Within a few years, these broths came to be called "Coley's toxins." And for several decades, they were used extensively—until medical science turned to radiation and chemotherapies, and the clinical use of bacterial cultures was abandoned.

But Coley's toxins were not entirely forgotten. A number of researchers retained an interest in the unexplained effect of bacterial infections on cancer. Coley himself had written in 1891, "Nature often gives us hints to her profoundest secrets, and it is possible that she has given us a hint which, if we will but follow, may lead us on to the solution of this difficult problem."*

Four decades after he wrote those words, researchers began to investigate nature's hint to see what it might reveal.

In one important experiment, guinea pigs were inoculated with tumor cells, which eventually formed visible nodules on

*Coley, W. B. 1891. Contribution to the knowledge of sarcoma. *Ann. Surg.* 14: 199–220.

the skin. Researchers then injected the animals with an active bacterial culture broth. Within four hours, the central portion of each tumor mass had begun to darken, the result of hemorraging. Tumor cells began to die, and within a short time the tumor itself was sloughed off. Curiously, although a large portion of the tumor was destroyed in the process, an outer ring of tumor cells remained. And these cancer cells began to grow again, eventually creating a new tumor.

In 1944, J. M. Shear, a researcher at the National Cancer Institute, discovered the active factor in the antitumor bacterial broths. Coley's toxins were in fact endotoxins—the substances from bacterial cell walls that would later be found to trigger macrophages to release interleukin 1. When investigators injected purified endotoxins into animals with large skin tumors, the cells of the tumors quickly began to hemorrhage. The blackened tissue, containing coagulated blood and dead tumor cells, eventually separated from the underlying tissue and was sloughed off.

Understandably excited by these experiments, researchers added the purified endotoxins directly to cultures of tumor cells. The results both surprised and puzzled them. The tumor cells continued to grow, totally unaffected by the very substances that would doom them in a living animal.

Only one conclusion could be made. Endotoxins must work indirectly on tumor cells in animals. They must somehow act through an intermediary, triggering host cells or substances, which in turn are responsible for destroying the tumor cells. But exactly what this intermediary was and how it worked remained a mystery for thirty years—until 1975, when E. A. Carswell and his colleagues at the Memorial Sloan-Kettering Cancer Center discovered a new group of lymphokines at work.

Carswell and his research team began a series of experiments by injecting healthy mice with endotoxins and collecting the blood serum several hours later. A portion of the serum was then injected into other mice that had already developed observable tumors. Within hours, the cancer cells began to die, and within a week the central portions of the tumors had fallen away. Residual amounts of toxin in the serum were much too low to account for this effect. And unlike endotoxins, the antitumor serum was also able to destroy tumor cells in laboratory dishes. The experiment provided the first direct evidence that endotoxins, introduced into the body, stimulated the release of another substance into the bloodstream—a substance capable of destroying tumor cells. Scientists called this substance *tumor necrosis factor.*

Immunologists have determined that tumor necrosis factor is clearly distinct from interleukin 1, interleukin 2, and migration inhibitory factor. It is indeed a new and unique lymphokine—perhaps even a group of lymphokines. Today, many researchers believe that tumor necrosis factor is produced by macrophages. In a laboratory dish, macrophages stimulated with endotoxin will produce one or more lymphokines that cause tumor cells to die. Injected into laboratory animals, the broth from macrophage cultures will also attack and kill tumor cells.

A great many questions remain. Researchers do not understand, for example, how tumor necrosis factor differentiates between normal and cancerous cells. And this group of lymphokines appears to be effective in targeting only certain kinds of tumor cells; we do not yet understand why.

But beyond these specific questions, research on tumor necrosis factor has raised a more fundamental question—one that may have far-reaching implications. The activity of tumor necrosis factor suggests an important relationship between the immune system's response to bacterial infection and the control of emerging cancer cells within the body. A powerful immune response against certain kinds of bacterial infections seems to have a secondary, but critical defense role: the elimination of developing tumor cells. As long ago as 1944, J. M. Shear, the researcher who first isolated the active principle of Coley's toxins, understood the startling and troublesome implications of these discoveries. "Are pathogenic and non-pathogenic organisms one of Nature's controls of . . . malignant disease," he wrote, "and, in making progress in the control of infectious diseases, are we removing one of Nature's controls of cancer?"*

There is little doubt that the incidence of cancer has risen dramatically in the last forty years, a period during which antibiotics have profoundly diminished the incidence of serious bacterial infections. Most researchers have accepted the hypothesis that the rise in cancer is, in large part, the result of a substantial increase in environmental pollutants and food additives. But it may well be that the rise in cancer is also the result of a decrease in major bacterial infections. By controlling these infections therapeutically, we may have inadvertently robbed the immune system of a powerful mechanism for the control of tumor cells.

Since the discovery of migration inhibitory factor, less than twenty years ago, immunologists have made giant steps forward in understanding the role lymphokines play in immune responses. We now know that a variety of different lymphokines

---

*J. M. Shear: see discussion of paper by Reinhard, E. J., J. T. Good, and E. Martin. 1950. Chemotherapy of malignant neoplastic diseases. *JAMA* 142:383–390.

control every growth and functional response of each and every cell engaged in the body's defense. B cells reproduce and manufacture antibody because helper T cells release specific lymphokines that signal them to do so. Cells migrate toward the site of an immune response because other cells already there release lymphokines, called *chemotactic factors,* which possess the ability to attract distant cells where and when they are needed. Whenever a circulating phagocyte or lymphocyte makes contact with a specific chemotactic factor, it will migrate toward the source of that factor. The more chemotactic factor an immune cell comes in contact with, the more rapidly the cell moves toward its source—the site of an infection or inflammation. After immune responses have successfully defended the body against attack, suppressor T cells release specific lymphokines that issue the equivalent of a cease-fire command. These lymphokines are able to turn off particular immune cells when the job of defense is done.

Immune responsiveness is in fact a complex network of immune cell interactions mediated by a wide range of lymphokines. Each cell issues its own commands by releasing specific lymphokines, and each cell responds to the commands of other cells by interpreting their lymphokine signals. As the body alters its strategies for defense, the measure and balance of lymphokines shifts delicately. When the majority of lymphokine signals come from interleukin 1 and interleukin 2, for example, immune cells are driven to the peak of their activity. But as lymphokines released by suppressor T cells begin to shift the balance, immune cells cease their activity, and the body's immune response comes to an end.

As immunologists have deciphered the powerful language of lymphokines, they have wondered at the possibility of harnessing the power of these substances to control and direct immune responses therapeutically. Could lymphokines like interleukin 1, interleukin 2, and tumor necrosis factor one day be used as drugs to help the body in its fight against disease?

Ironically, the story of lymphokine therapy begins not with the discovery of lymphokines, but with chicken eggs, viruses, and a substance that was first identified several years before migration inhibitory factor. This substance has gradually revealed the full range of its extraordinary powers. Its name is interferon.

five

THE PROMISE OF LYMPHOKINES

It's time to bite the bullet on interferon.

FRANK RAUSCHER

In 1957, a revolutionary scientific paper appeared in the *Proceedings of the Royal Society of London,* quietly sandwiched between a report on bacterial growth in the presence of antibiotics and another on the social behavior of honeybees.

Researchers Alick Isaacs and Jean Lindenmann had set out to unravel a small but compelling mystery. When inactivated viruses were added to cultures of living embryonic chicken cells, they somehow protected the cells from attack by other active viruses. At first Isaacs and Lindenmann had supposed that the viruses, by binding harmlessly to the cells, protected them from being bound by active and potentially destructive viruses. The results of several preliminary experiments argued against this idea, however. So the researchers tried another experiment. They placed the embryonic cells in culture with inactive viruses for two hours and then washed the viruses away. When active viruses were later added to this culture, Isaacs and Lindenmann were surprised to find that the cells were still protected from attack, even though the inactive viruses had been completely removed. These startling results seemed to prove that inactivated viruses did not themselves protect the cells. Instead, the inactivated viruses appeared to stimulate the cells to produce a substance which, secreted into the local environment, protected them from attack. Because this newly identified substance interfered with the activity of viruses, Isaacs and Lindenmann called it *interferon.*

The discovery of interferon had enormous implications. No other substance had ever been observed to protect cells against an invading virus. That interferon occurred naturally, the result of contact between a virus and the body's cells, suggested a powerful strategy for defense. With a tremendous sense of excitement, researchers around the world set about to uncover the nature and function of interferon.

Today we know that interferon is not a single substance but at least a dozen related proteins, each able to block viruses from infecting cells. The many forms of interferon have been divided into three major chemical groups: *alpha, beta,* and *gamma* interferon. Among these, there are at least eight forms of alpha interferon, three types of beta, and one of gamma interferon.

Alpha and beta interferon were the first to be identified and tested. Researchers discovered that many types of cells within the body, including immune cells as well as the cells that make up tissues and organs, can produce alpha and beta interferon. Inactive and active viruses, as well as chemical substances secreted by certain fungi and bacteria, can stimulate interferon production. Cells release alpha and beta interferon into the local environment, where these protein molecules bind to nearby healthy cells, protecting them from fatal encounters with the invading pathogens. Alpha and beta interferon somehow prevent viruses from using a cell's materials and machinery for reproduction, but how this is accomplished is not yet clearly understood. The remarkable fact about interferon is that it can block an invading virus from commandeering the cell's protein synthesis machinery even while it allows the cell to go on conducting its own synthesizing processes.

Gamma interferon, like alpha and beta, can protect cells from viral attack. But in most other ways it is unique. Gamma interferon is produced by only one kind of cell, an activated T cell engaged in an immune response; it is therefore the only true lymphokine among the different groups of interferon. Its role in the body's defense is far-reaching. In fact, investigators have discovered that gamma interferon is a critical component in the battle against almost every one of the body's enemies—viruses, bacteria, fungi, and protozoa alike.

Experiments with an unusually lethal group of bacteria and protozoa gave immunologists compelling evidence of the extraordinary powers of gamma interferon. Most bacteria and protozoa are engulfed and destroyed by phagocytes. But certain of these pathogens—those that cause tuberculosis, leprosy, and African sleeping sickness, for example—are somehow able to protect themselves from being destroyed even after they have been engulfed by a phagocyte. These pathogens can actually colonize the very cells that were designed to destroy them, growing until the phagocytes themselves are destroyed.

On their own, phagocytes are helpless against these pathogens. But in the presence of T cells, they somehow gain the ability to destroy the invading bacteria and protozoa. Researchers considered it unlikely that T cells were directly involved in this destruction, simply because a primary attack against the colonizing pathogens would destroy the phagocytes as well. It seemed far more likely that T cells were in some way activating a special killing mechanism within the phagocytes themselves. Researchers began to wonder if T cells offered their help to phagocytes in the form of a lymphokine.

To find out, they infected a culture of phagocytes with protozoa, which quickly colonized the helpless immune cells. Using a microscope, researchers could actually count the number of protozoa within each phagocyte. They knew that if T cells were added to the culture, the phagocytes would gain the ability to destroy the protozoa. Instead of directly adding T cells, however, the investigators added broth from a culture of T cells. Once again the original culture was placed under a microscope and examined for protozoa surviving within the phagocytes. The results were dramatic. The broth had worked just as effectively as the presence of T cells. Hardly a single protozoan remained.

Obviously T cells helped phagocytes defend themselves against invasion by secreting some sort of substance into the broth. But what was the precise nature of this substance? Had researchers discovered a new lymphokine, or simply a new activity of a previously known substance such as migration inhibitory factor or interleukin 2?

The first step in answering these questions was to separate

and purify the substance secreted by T cells. Once this substance was purified, researchers could compare it to other well-characterized lymphokines. Their findings would add a new chapter to the dramatic story of interferon. The substance that helped phagocytes destroy invading bacteria and protozoa was gamma interferon.

And before long, additional experiments demonstrated that the role of gamma interferon in immune responses was even more complex. Researchers discovered that gamma interferon, injected into a culture of macrophages, stimulates these cells to produce interleukin 1. Interleukin 1 then triggers T cells to produce interleukin 2, as we've seen, which causes T cells to grow in number and to release migration inhibitory factor. Interleukin 2 also stimulates T cells to release another substance: gamma interferon.

A new lymphokine cycle had been identified, one that helps to amplify and expand the body's defense against infection by increasing the number of active macrophages and T cells participating in a specific immune response.

Intrigued by the surprising range of gamma interferon's powers, a group of investigators devised an elegant experiment to test its potential function in fighting cancer. Their experiment was designed to measure not the *direct* effect of gamma interferon but rather its *absence* from an immune response against cancer. The researchers already knew that when laboratory mice were inoculated with tumor cells, their spleens would later be found to contain large numbers of killer T cells capable of attacking and destroying the tumors. But no one knew what triggered the generation of these killer T cells. Could gamma interferon play a role?

The investigators began by preparing an antibody that

would target and neutralize any gamma interferon produced in the cultures, effectively blocking whatever role it might play in either the stimulation of killer T cells or their attack against tumor cells. When these antibodies were injected into culture dishes containing spleen cells and tumor cells, the results were dramatic. In the cultures where gamma interferon remained active, killer T cells attacked and destroyed every one of the tumor cells. In the cultures that contained antibodies against interferon, no active killer T cells were observed, and the tumor cells were flourishing.

The experiment proved that gamma interferon, part of the lymphokine cycle that involves interleukin 1 and interleukin 2, is a necessary component in the production of active killer T cells. Investigators later determined that gamma interferon functions by initiating the final stage in the activation of killer T cells. Without the presence of this lymphokine, cells destined to become killer T cells grow but never develop the ability to seek out and destroy either virally invaded cells or tumor cells. Gamma interferon also appears to work in the body's defense against cancer in another way—by stimulating natural killer cells to attack and destroy tumor cells.

With each new insight into interferon and its powers, hopes ran high that this potent substance would prove to be nothing short of a wonder drug. After all, interferon in the laboratory could protect cells against viral attack. Even more amazing, interferon seemed to enhance the body's defense against cancer. Medical science possesses very few weapons against either forms of disease. And here was a naturally occurring protein, part of the body's own defense system, which promised to offer help in the battle against both.

The first clinical tests of interferon were conducted with cancer patients, beginning in the early 1970s. Only the antiviral activities of interferon were known at the time (gamma interferon, the true lymphokine, had yet to be characterized). But there was still reason to hope that the antiviral properties of alpha and beta interferon would make them effective against cancer cells. Animal studies had clearly demonstrated that certain kinds of cancer were caused by viruses that could transform normal cells into tumor cells. And although the exact role of viruses in human cancer was highly controversial (and remains so even today), it seemed possible that interferon might be of significant value in the treatment of cancer in humans.

From the very beginning, there were severe limitations on the testing of interferon. Only very small quantities of alpha and beta interferon were available for use with patients, and this lack of sufficient quantities of the drug hampered researchers. To be effective in the body, a drug, whether aspirin or interferon, must be present at an optimal concentration. If the drug level falls below a critical concentration, the patient does not benefit from its potential therapeutic effect. Conversely, if the concentration rises beyond a certain point, toxic side effects may occur. So little interferon existed at the time of the early studies that researchers had no way to determine proper dosages and schedules for the treatment of specific types of cancer. No one knew how much interferon to administer, when to administer it, or even how the drug should be administered. In some studies, in fact, researchers ran out of interferon before the studies could be completed. Clinical trials were initiated with precious little interferon and very small groups of cancer patients, most of whom were already in a terminal state of the illness. Interferon was their last hope.

The early results were disappointing. Although certain studies reported decreased tumor size and short-term remissions after interferon treatment, there was no definite evidence that any patient had been cured of cancer by the drug. And the high hopes for interferon seemed to fall with each new clinical study. In March 1980, *Time* magazine asked, "Will the natural drug interferon fulfill its early promise?" As recently as 1983, the *Journal of the American Medical Association* answered the question this way: "The honeymoon is over. After years of intensive study, cancer researchers are no longer making glowing predictions about interferon's anticancer effects."

Still, that judgment may one day be revised. After a decade of research, the clinical study of interferon is really still in its infancy. Only very recently have researchers been able to use recombinant DNA technology to produce large quantities of purified alpha, beta, and gamma interferon for clinical use. And clinicians are already reporting promising results from preliminary tests. New studies suggest that interferon may yet become a significant drug in the treatment of cancer—especially cancers resistant to conventional therapies.

Interferon appears to be effective against malignant melanoma, for example, a cancer of the pigmented skin cells that has proved extremely difficult to treat with conventional anticancer drugs. In a recent study of sixteen patients with malignant melanoma, two patients were in complete remission after ten months of interferon treatment, and five others were stabilized with no increase in tumor development. A similar study at the Mayo Clinic found three patients in complete remission after five to seven months of interferon therapy.

Interferon is also proving itself in the treatment of cancer of the kidney, another cancer that usually resists conventional chemotherapies. In a new study at the Memorial Sloan-Kettering Cancer Center, investigators found that ten of thirty-three patients with kidney cancer were responding well to interferon therapy. In five of those patients, tumor size was diminished by at least 50 percent. In the past, conventional drug therapy had produced, at best, only a 10 percent decrease in the size of kidney tumors.

The therapeutic potential of interferon in the treatment of other cancers, including breast cancer, colon cancer, and leukemia, is still under investigation. Although no complete cures have been observed, a significant number of patients have shown clinical improvement—sufficient improvement to warrant further studies with interferon. Many researchers are now confident that interferon will become a useful form of therapy for a number of cancers, perhaps in conjunction with one or more conventional anticancer drugs.

Popular interest has always focused on the potential of interferon as a wonder drug for cancer. But apart from the headlines and news briefs, interferon is proving itself—less dramatically, perhaps, but no less significantly—as a highly effective drug in the treatment of certain viral diseases. Indeed, the major therapeutic use of interferon in the future may well be in the control of viral infections.

Clinicians at the Karolinska Institute in Stockholm, for example, have been studying the effects of interferon on papilloma viruses. These viruses cause benign growths on the skin called papillomas or warts. In most cases, warts pose no serious health problem. But in some instances they can occur on the vocal cords, occasionally filling up the entire larynx and severely impairing breathing. In children, the condition is usually treated by the surgical removal of the papillomas. But surgery cannot prevent their recurrence. And in some patients these growths may recur so quickly that surgery must be repeated again and again. One child afflicted with the disease required almost four hundred operations.

Frustrated by the inadequacies of surgery, investigators at the Karolinska Institute initiated interferon trials with a group of seven children. The results were dramatic and conclusive. In three of the children, the papillomas were entirely eliminated. In the other, more severe cases, fewer papillomas recurred after the children were placed on a maintenance dose of interferon.

Interferon is also providing protection against the onset of certain opportunistic infections in immunosuppressed transplant patients. Because of the high risk of rejection in transplant surgery, physicians routinely administer immunosuppressive drugs to block the activity of immune cells which would otherwise attack the transplanted tissue and destroy it. Unfortunately, these drugs leave transplant patients dangerously vulnerable to a wide variety of opportunistic infections. One of the most serious is cytomegalovirus infection. CMV infection can result in fever and a precipitous drop in white blood cells; and it can leave a transplant patient even more susceptible to secondary bacterial, fungal, or protozoal infections, kidney dysfunction, and certain kinds of cancer. At Massachusetts General Hospital in Boston, investigators are finding interferon to be effective in preventing the activation of latent cytomegaloviruses in transplant patients. Treatment with interferon before and after kidney transplant surgery not only decreases the incidence of cytomegalovirus infection, but significantly reduces the risk of secondary infection by other pathogens.

Interferon may even offer relief from the ravages of the common cold. While research indicates that interferon is not effective against colds already in progress, individuals given interferon intranasally and then exposed to the cold-causing rhinovirus have exhibited over a 90 percent reduction in the incidence of cold symptoms. Several pharmaceutical companies are already developing plans to market nasal preparations of interferon for prophylactic use against colds. But there are potential drawbacks to interferon use in nasal preparations. Prolonged exposure to interferon nasal sprays can cause nasal bleeding, which may ultimately prevent this form of interferon therapy from being widely accepted.

Throughout more than a decade of clinical interferon testing, in fact, researchers have been surprised by the broad range of side effects to the drug. At high doses, interferon can cause disorientation and seizures, as well as liver damage. Several patients, especially those with a history of heart disease, have developed severe cardiovascular problems during the course of treatment. Fortunately, these severe side effects have been rare. Most patients treated with interferon experience milder symptoms of fever, fatigue, loss of appetite, malaise, and chills. During the first testing of interferon, investigators assumed that the side effects were caused by a contaminating substance in the interferon preparations. But in the most recent studies, patients receiving pure preparations of recombinant DNA interferon have experienced the same symptoms. It now seems more likely that the side effects are caused by a fundamental immunologic activity of interferon: the stimulation of interleukin 1 production. As interferon enters the body, it may activate macrophages to produce increased levels of interleukin 1. Interleukin 1, released into the bloodstream, may then induce fever and the breakdown of muscle protein, causing the flu-like symptoms many patients experience after interferon treatments.

There is still much to be learned about how to administer interferon—in what dosages, and in what form. Gamma interferon is only now becoming available in sufficient quantities for clinical testing, and many researchers believe that this form of interferon may prove to be the most powerful of the three. There is even the possibility that certain combinations of alpha, beta, and gamma interferon may be more effective than any one form. (As one researcher has asked, "Why did God give you enough genes to make twelve different kinds of interferon if one was enough?")

Immunologists may eventually discover that the effectiveness of interferon is increased when used along with other lymphokines—tumor necrosis factor, for example, or interleukin 2. Tumor necrosis factor is an extremely powerful weapon against tumors, but for reasons not well understood, it leaves a ring of living cells even after it has destroyed the central core of a tumor. Used in conjunction with other lymphokines, however, tumor necrosis factor may make possible the total destruction of tumors. And the activities of interferon, and perhaps tumor necrosis factor as well, may be enhanced when administered along with another potent lymphokine: interleukin 2.

Investigators had their first glimpse into the extraordinary therapeutic potential of interleukin 2 during experiments with the special strain of mice known as nude mice. Since this strain is born without a functional thymus gland, nude mice survive without the help of immunologically active helper, killer, and suppressor T cells. When spleen cells from nude mice are placed in culture dishes and exposed to an antigen, they produce few if any antibodies. (Without the assistance of active helper T cells, B cells from nude mice lack the lymphokine signals that are absolutely essential if they are to grow into mature antibody secreting cells.)

Researchers already knew that, by adding mature helper T cells from normal mice to the spleen cell cultures, they could stimulate the B cells of nude mice to divide and eventually produce high levels of antibodies in response to the presence of foreign antigens. And a series of experiments demonstrated that one particular T cell lymphokine, interleukin 2, played a critical role in restoring these antibody responses. Although nude mice lack a functioning thymus, the gland in which T cells mature, they still produce bone marrow precursors of mature T cells. Researchers discovered that interleukin 2 is capable of stimulating the maturation of T cells that have never passed through the thymus. These precursors are then able to develop into fully functional helper T cells, which release two lymphokines that act directly on B cells to induce the production of antibodies.

Intrigued by these initial observations on interleukin 2, researchers began to wonder if an injection of this lymphokine could restore other immune responses deficient in nude mice. They knew, for example, that this strain also lacks mature killer T cells. Could interleukin 2 restore the function of killer T cells? To find out, researchers injected tumor cells into cultures of immune cells from nude mice. Untreated, the immune cells were completely unable to respond to the tumor cells. But when researchers added interleukin 2 to the culture, killer T cells actively attacked and destroyed the tumors.

These twin findings were nothing short of astonishing. Interleukin 2, a single protein molecule, had replaced a complete biologic function normally associated with an entire organ, the thymus. Interleukin 2 obviously possessed extraordinary potency in a laboratory dish. But would it reconstitute T cell function in living laboratory mice?

The experiment was simple. Two groups of nude mice were injected with tumor cells, but only one set received interleukin 2. After several days, researchers examined spleens taken from both groups for the presence of killer T cells. The spleens of the untreated nude mice contained no killer T cells at all, but the spleens of those mice injected with interleukin 2 contained a fully functional population of killer T cells. The experiment proved that interleukin 2 is not simply a laboratory curiosity, but a highly potent lymphokine capable of restoring immunologic activity in living animals. And researchers soon discovered that interleukin 2 possesses another important ability. Injected into a culture of immune cells, interleukin 2 stimulates the growth of natural killer cells—the cells that are believed to be a major weapon in the body's defense against both virally infected cells and tumor cells.

With these findings, researchers began to wonder whether interleukin 2, by increasing the numbers of killer T cells and natural killer cells in the body, might substantially strengthen an immune response against a tumor or invading virus. To test that possibility, they conceived a unique therapeutic technique. The first step would involve isolating a cancer patient's own T cells and natural killer cells, and then culturing them in laboratory dishes containing interleukin 2, which would stimulate the immune cells to reproduce. These new cells could then be injected into the patient, giving the immune system additional forces with which to destroy the original tumor.

This potential therapy has already been tested successfully in laboratory mice. A group of mice were injected with tumor cells in order to generate the production of killer T cells in their spleens. After several days, the killer T cells were removed and grown in a culture broth containing interleukin 2. Interleukin 2 stimulated the growth and development of large numbers of killer T cells. Researchers then inoculated a second group of mice with tumors cells. Several of these infected mice were injected with the killer T cells cultured with interleukin 2. The results were striking. The animals that did not receive injections of killer T cells died within a short time after being inoculated with tumor cells. The other mice, injected with killer T cells stimulated by interleukin 2, exhibited dramatically increased survival times.

Researchers at the National Institutes of Health have now begun to study the possible use of this therapy in cancer patients. These experiments may well confirm the effectiveness of the technique; but many investigators still doubt its practical benefits. It may simply prove impossible, both from a technical and economic standpoint, to isolate and grow T cells and natural killer cells for the tens of thousands of cancer patients who might benefit from the therapy. Many researchers believe that a more practical use of interleukin 2 in cancer patients may be by direct injection, perhaps in conjunction with some form of interferon. And studies are now underway to explore the effectiveness of such therapy.

There is hope that interleukin 2 may prove effective in patients with various immunodeficiency diseases as well. These diseases are marked by the breakdown or absence of one or more components of normal immune responses. In Nezelof's syndrome, for example, the population of T cells is severely depressed or absent, leaving victims of the disease susceptible to a wide variety of infections. Recently, investigators at Memorial Sloan-Kettering Cancer Center discovered that T cells from a three-year-old patient with Nezelof's syndrome were unable to produce interleukin 2. When they supplemented the patient's T cells with interleukin 2 from another source, however, the cells regained their normal responsiveness. Experiments are currently underway to test the effectiveness of interleukin 2 in restoring immune responses in patients with Acquired Immune Deficiency Syndrome.

Immunologists are also interested in testing the clinical potential of interleukin 1. Ironically, this lymphokine is so potent, affecting so many different kinds of cells, that its usefulness in stimulating immune responses may be limited. Interleukin 1 stimulates T cells to produce interleukin 2, but it also triggers fever and the muscular ache and weakness commonly associated with an infection. Because of these side effects, the future importance of interleukin 1 in clinical therapy may be based not on directly administering the lymphokine but on *blocking* its activity in the body.

Investigators have recently discovered that a number of arthritic and lung diseases are associated with excessive production of interleukin 1. The symptoms of chronic inflammatory diseases like rheumatoid arthritis, for example, may actually result, at least in part, from uncontrolled interleukin 1 production. In studies at Massachusetts General Hospital, investigators were able to isolate a population of specialized cells, called *synovial cells,* from the joints of patients with rheumatoid arthritis. These cells are capable of producing copious amounts of two substances known to be involved in the destruction of joint tissue. And in a collaborative effort with researchers at the National Institutes of Health, investigators found that synovial cells were stimulated by interleukin 1.

That discovery has suggested the possibility of a unique form of therapy. If researchers can learn to *block* the action of interleukin 1, using natural or synthetic fragments of interleukin 1 that are called *antagonists,* they may be able to control the destructive activities of synovial cells—and stop the debilitating tissue damage caused by certain inflammatory diseases.

The extraordinary progress in lymphokine research and the therapeutic testing of lymphokines has astonished even many scientists. Important discoveries are being made not year by year, but month by month, and even week by week. And the pace is accelerating. Almost ten years elapsed between the initial discovery of interleukin 1 and interleukin 2 and their eventual purification and chemical characterization. Fewer than three years passed before researchers, using recombinant DNA techniques, were able to transfer the genes for interleukin 2 into bacteria capable of producing large amounts of the powerful lymphokine. And within a few months, interleukin 2 was being tested in patients with Acquired Immune Deficiency Syndrome.

Indeed, the dramatic appearance of this new and lethal disease has brought a sharpened sense of urgency to lymphokine research. Desperately struggling to treat the disease, immunologists have already experimented extensively with interferon. And clinical tests are currently underway to evaluate the effect of interleukin 2 in restoring immune responses in AIDS patients. In the future, as yet unidentified lymphokines may come to play important roles in treating not only Acquired

Immune Deficiency Syndrome, but the wide range of other immune deficiency diseases—diseases which leave their victims virtually defenseless against the assault of the body's microbial enemies.

six

OUT OF AMMUNITION

For it has been found in almost all things that what they contained [that] is useful and applicable, is hardly ever perceived unless we are deprived of them.

WILLIAM HARVEY (1578–1657)

In 1951, Ogden Bruton, a physician at Walter Reed Army Hospital in Washington, D.C., examined an eight-year-old boy with a serious bacterial infection and a troubling medical history. During the previous five years, the boy had developed at least twenty severe infections, most of which had vigorously resisted conventional treatment. Even more disturbing, all attempts to vaccinate the young patient had failed. He was seriously ill, and no one knew exactly why.

Searching for a clue, Bruton examined the protein makeup of the boy's blood, and what he discovered astounded him. The young patient appeared to have no antibodies circulating in his bloodstream. It was as if the boy possessed no humoral immunity at all.

Shortly after Bruton released his findings, several physicians in Boston contacted him, reporting that they too had treated other young patients whose blood showed the same abnormality: a low or undetectable level of antibodies. And during the next five years, over forty cases of the rare condition—called *agammaglobulinemia* (no detectable antibodies) or *hypogammaglobulinemia* (abnormally low levels of antibodies)—were reported in the medical literature. Immunologic tests indicated that patients with the two rare diseases possess few if any mature B cells—the basic cellular machinery for the production of antibodies. In some patients, immature B cells seem to be unable to develop into antibody-producing cells. Other patients lack altogether the bone marrow cells that give rise to B cells. Symptoms of the two diseases usually appear five to six months after birth, when maternal antibodies transferred to the fetus have essentially disappeared from the newborn's circulation (and when, in normal individuals, the developing B cell population begins to produce its own antibodies). As maternal antibodies disappear, patients with the rare disease syndrome begin to develop various infections, including pneumonia and other infections of the upper and lower respiratory tract.

Bruton's diagnosis of agammaglobulinemia in his eight-year-old patient was a major landmark in clinical medicine. For the first time, researchers had recognized a disease whose cause was a fundamental deficiency of the body's immune system—the very system whose job was to defend against disease. And in the years that followed, as new and more sophisticated immunologic tests made it possible to analyze the activity of separate components of the immune system, researchers identified a wide range of diseases that result from specific deficiencies of one or more of the cells or substances involved in immune responses, disorders of T and B cell function, phagocyte activity, antibody synthesis, complement production—in fact, deficiencies of any one of virtually *every* component of the immune system have been identified.

Ironically, the study of immunodeficiency diseases has provided a unique window into the workings of the healthy immune system. Since each type of immunodeficiency disease is associated with a specific immunologic defect or dysfunction, researchers can observe, in its absence or dysfunction, the critical importance of the altered or absent immune component in the overall network of immune responses. By studying the failure of the body to produce a specific class of antibodies —immunoglobulin A, for example—researchers have had a clearer view of how IgA works in a fully functioning immune system. Patients with IgA deficiencies (one of the most common forms of immunodeficiency) experience a higher incidence of respiratory infections, confirming the fact that IgA, found in body secretions, plays an important role in defending the exposed surfaces of the body against attack. Researchers have found that IgA-deficient patients also have a high incidence of asthma and allergy—suggesting, perhaps, that the absence of IgA allows antigens to reach sites in the respiratory tract, where they can induce asthmatic or allergic symptoms.

A wide variety of immunodeficiencies are congenital, the result of primary defects in the cells or cell substances of the immune system. But immunologists have also identified secondary immunodeficiencies, conditions in which immune responsiveness is suppressed by external factors. As long ago as 1908, immunologists observed that certain pathogenic organisms are able to suppress immune responses. Mumps and measles viruses, for example, as well as the bacteria responsible for tuberculosis and leprosy, can subvert and disable the immune system during an infection. In some viruses, the proteins that surround the viral genetic material seem to have the ability to suppress immune responses in laboratory animals or in cultures of immune cells, "turning off" the activities of both macrophages and T cells. Fortunately their effect is transient. Once the primary infection is resolved, the secondary effect of immunosuppression ends. Malnutrition can also cause a secondary state of immunosuppression. Without adequate protein and caloric intake, the body's immune defense mechanisms become severely impaired. The thymus gland loses its ability to produce T cells, leaving the victims of malnutrition prey to a wide variety of opportunistic infections.

Secondary immunosuppression is also a troublesome and sometimes serious side effect of certain drug therapies. Most of the drugs used in the treatment of cancer drastically suppress immune responses. The targets of such therapy are tumor cells, of course; but anticancer drugs are not specific. They block the growth of all fast-growing cells, including lymphocytes. (Many of the same drugs are used in transplant patients specifically to destroy immune cells and thereby prevent the rejection of grafted organs or tissue.) Patients undergoing chemotherapy become dangerously susceptible to a number of opportunistic infections. Like the effect of certain pathogens, the immunosuppression caused by anticancer drugs is transient. Once chemotherapy is concluded, immune responsiveness returns to normal.

In severely burned patients, virtually *all* immune functions are seriously depressed, including the level of antibodies circulating in the blood, the activity of phagocytes, and the number and activity of T cells. Immunologists do not fully understand the underlying cause of these severe changes in immune responsiveness, but their consequences are well documented. Infections are the leading cause of death in burn patients.

Over the past thirty years, then, researchers have identified and characterized a spectrum of immunodeficiencies—some the result of congenital defects in immune components, others the secondary effects of primary factors like malnutrition or immunosuppressive drug therapies. More recently, epidemiologists and immunologists have charted the emergence of a new and lethal immunodeficiency syndrome, one very different in its nature from any that had been observed before: a severe acquired immunodeficiency syndrome that appears to be transmitted by an infectious organism.

Early in 1981, a young man entered New York University hospital complaining of prolonged fever and severe, unexplained weight loss. The patient's spleen was abnormally enlarged and his lymph nodes swollen. Examining physicians noticed several reddish-purple spots on the skin of the patient's legs, but these were assumed to be nothing more than bruises. When dermatologist Alvin Friedman-Kien examined the young man, however, the spots caught his attention. They resembled the lesions of an extremely rare skin cancer called Kaposi's sarcoma, a form of cancer seen almost exclusively among men in their sixties and seventies and in patients receiving immunosuppressive drugs—and even then only rarely. The incidence of Kaposi's sarcoma in the United States is only 1 in 2,500,000. The mean age of patients affected by it is sixty-three. A diagnosis of the disease in a young man would be highly unusual.

Still, Friedman-Kien ordered a biopsy of the patient's lesions. His first impression had been right: the lesions were indeed Kaposi's sarcoma.

During the same period, physicians at the Medical Center of University of California at Los Angeles examined a thirty-one-year-old man with a severe fungal infection of the throat. The patient had suffered drastic weight loss during the past several months, along with unexplained fevers and swollen lymph nodes. Immunologist Michael S. Gottlieb, searching for the cause of these severe symptoms, was puzzled. Uncontrolled fungal infections of the sort he had diagnosed usually indicated a breakdown of the immune system. But the patient didn't seem to fit into any known immune disorder, and Gottlieb was unable to identify any external factors that might be responsible for a state of immunosuppression. Within two weeks, however, the patient went on to develop the rare lung infection called *Pneumocystis* pneumonia, a lethal disease seen almost exclusively in cancer or transplant patients receiving immunosuppressive drugs.

And at almost the same time, a young man entered the University of California Medical Center in San Francisco, alarmed at the sudden appearance of several reddish-purple spots on his skin. Examining physicians ordered a biopsy of the unusual skin lesions. The diagnosis: the rare skin cancer called Kaposi's sarcoma. The case might have been an anomaly. But within a matter of months, a growing number of cases of Kaposi's sarcoma, *Pneumocystis* pneumonia, and other rare opportunistic infections were diagnosed in San Francisco. And all of the patients there, as well as in New York and Los Angeles, had at least one provocative thing in common: they were all young male homosexuals.

On June 5, 1981, the first report of a new and alarming disease syndrome appeared in the Center for Disease Control's *Morbidity and Mortality Weekly Report.* Five young homosexual men had been treated in Los Angeles hospitals for *Pneumocystis carinii* pneumonia and other rare infections. Two of the young men were dead. "*Pneumocystis* pneumonia in the United States is almost exclusively limited to severely immunosuppressed patients," the report stated. "The occurrence of pneumocystosis in 5 previously healthy individuals without a clinically apparent underlying immunodefiency is unusual."

By the time the report appeared, however, the disease was no longer so unusual. More than twenty gay men in New York City and six in California had been diagnosed with either Kaposi's sarcoma or *Pneumocystis* pneumonia—and eight of the patients had died.

In June 1981, the Centers for Disease Control began the systematic surveillance of what was being called Acquired Immune Deficiency Syndrome, or AIDS. A special task force gathered reports of previously healthy patients between the ages of fifteen and sixty who had developed either Kaposi's sarcoma or life-threatening opportunistic infections. As the weeks and months passed, the number of reported cases of the devastating syndrome increased alarmingly. Since the second half of 1979, when the first cases of the disease were believed to have appeared, the incidence of AIDS was doubling every six months. In September 1982, more than two cases were reported to the CDC every day; by March 1983, six months later, an average of four to five cases of AIDS were being tallied daily.

By then it was clear not only that a new disease syndrome

had appeared, but that it was already reaching epidemic proportions. And investigators had virtually no idea what caused it.

During the first year of investigation of AIDS, the most compelling clue epidemiologists had to go on was the fact that virtually all its victims appeared to be gay men. Some investigators proposed that the disease might be caused by certain inhalant drugs frequently used by a number of these men—drugs called amyl and butyl nitrite, or "poppers." Because initial studies indicated that many of the patients had histories of sexual promiscuity, other researchers suggested that repeated exposure to sperm cells, which is known to have an immunosuppressive effect, might be the cause. As late as March 1982, during a special Public Health Service meeting on AIDS, both of these hypotheses were still being discussed with interest as possible causes of the disease.

But by then the epidemiological picture was already changing significantly, ruling out certain explanations, suggesting others, providing more clues—and more puzzlement. In the fall of 1981, New York physicians diagnosed AIDS in several heterosexual intravenous drugs users. During the same period, investigators in New York and New Jersey identified AIDS among a group of prisoners. Reports from New York and Florida confirmed the diagnosis of AIDS in several Haitians. And in the first months of 1982, investigators reported that a number of patients with hemophilia who regularly received blood transfusions had contracted the disease.

By August 1983, more than two thousand cases of AIDS had been confirmed. By then the groups most clearly at risk had been delineated. More than 70 percent of the patients were homosexual or bisexual men. Intravenous drug abusers accounted for 17 percent. One percent were patients with hemophilia, and 11 percent were Haitians, sexual partners of individuals within the other risk categories, or individuals who had received blood or blood products within the previous five years. What could gay men, intravenous drug abusers, Haitians, and hemophiliacs have in common that placed them at risk?

Epidemiologists, comparing the spread of this new disease syndrome with other known diseases, began to see a pattern. All four groups had one important thing in common: they were all high-risk groups for contracting the viral infection hepatitis B. Hepatitis B is communicated through sexual contact, which makes sexually active gay men particularly susceptible to it. Hepatitis B is also spread through exposure to blood products contaminated with the virus, placing both hemophiliacs and intravenous drug abusers at risk. The Haitian connection remained puzzling, although some epidemiologists suggested that there was evidence that the Haitians who had developed AIDS had engaged in homosexual activities, and might well have contracted the disease through sexual contact.

A frightening possibility was taking shape. Could the cause of AIDS, like the cause of hepatitis B, be a pathogenic organism? Could AIDS be an entirely new and terribly frightening kind of disease—a communicable immunodeficiency syndrome?

New evidence began to confirm that suspicion. Investigators turned up a cluster of gay men in Los Angeles, all of whom had in common at least one sexual partner, and all of whom had gone on, within the eighteen months that followed sexual contact, to develop Acquired Immune Deficiency Syndrome. In San Francisco, physicians diagnosed AIDS in an infant who had received blood transfusions shortly after birth. Searching the records of blood donors, they found that some of the transfused blood had been donated by a man who later developed the symptoms of AIDS (and had since died of the disease). The Centers for Disease Control received the report of AIDS in a woman who was the sexual partner of a man with AIDS. Evidence was growing that AIDS might indeed be caused by a communicable disease organism—something spread either by sexual contact or by exposure to contaminated blood products.

The clinical objectivity of these findings did not mask their frightening implications. If the disease was indeed communicable, it represented a serious public health emergency. More than one-half of the patients stricken were dead by the end of the first year; three years after onset of AIDS, virtually all of its victims had succumbed to the relentless succession of opportunistic infections. AIDS appeared to have the highest case fatality rate of virtually any disease known to man. Certainly it was one of the most lethal of all known immunodeficiency diseases. There was no evidence that anyone diagnosed with the disease had ever recovered.

And there was another disturbing fact. Epidemiological evidence had begun to suggest that AIDS had an unusually long latency period between the time of infection and the onset of symptoms—as long as two years, some investigators guessed. In one case, a Haitian man reportedly developed AIDS four years after receiving a blood transfusion that may have carried the disease organism. Such a long latency period was troubling for two reasons. The number of diagnosed cases of AIDS would then represent only a fraction of the number of individuals who had actually been infected, many of whom had yet to display the symptoms. And if the disease was transmissible, as many investigators had come to believe, individuals who had been infected but who had yet to show symptoms could be unknowingly infecting others.

On December 10, 1981, the *New England Journal of Medicine* published the results of three independent clinical studies involving nineteen patients. The patients all exhibited similar symptoms: recurrent fever, excessive weight loss, malaise, and one or more life-threatening opportunistic infections, including multiple viral infections, severe fungal infections, *Pneumocystis* pneumonia, and, in some cases, Kaposi's sarcoma.

Clinically, the nature of the illnesses associated with AIDS had already suggested to most researchers that the disease represented a severe breakdown of cell-mediated immunity. The injection of antigens under the skin of these patients did not evoke delayed-type hypersensitivity reactions—a sign that cell-mediated immunity was impaired. Laboratory tests confirmed these findings. Healthy T cells placed in culture with antigens proliferate and express their immune functions; but when T cells from AIDS patients were exposed to antigens, they failed to respond. The total number of lymphocyte cells was found to be abnormally low in all AIDS patients, and the proportion of helper T cells to other immune cells was far lower than normal. In most individuals there are two or three times as many helper T cells as suppressor T cells. But among AIDS patients, tests indicated far fewer helper cells than suppressor cells.

At the National Institutes of Health, Dr. Anthony Fauci and his co-workers found that cell-mediated immunity was not the only form of immune defense impaired in these patients. Abnormally high levels of all types of immunoglobulins were also found in blood samples of many AIDS patients. Some of these were autoantibodies—antibodies directed against the body's own cells. Paradoxically, laboratory tests demonstrated that the B cells of AIDS patients were unable to make antibody against specific antigens. Some unknown factor was stimulating the immune system to produce a wide range of nonspecific antibodies, while at the same time it impaired the normal production of antibodies in response to an antigen.

Some investigators argued that the B cell abnormalities found in AIDS patients might be a primary cause of the immune dysfunction, as they are in certain other immunodeficiency syndromes. But most investigators began to believe that the B cell abnormalities observed in AIDS are secondary to the suppression of T cell functions. Lymphokines produced by T cells are required not only for macrophage activation but also for B cell growth and the stimulation of antibody production. Without those activating lymphokines, B cell activities would be seriously undermined. By attacking the body's T cell population, the disease agent responsible for AIDS could set off a devastating chain reaction that would inexorably disrupt almost all parts of the immune system.

As the number of cases of AIDS rose, the search for its cause intensified. The special nature of AIDS as an immunodeficiency disease made that search particularly difficult. The epidemiologic profile of the disease left little doubt that the cause was an infectious organism, and most likely a virus. Unfortunately, AIDS patients are susceptible to a wide variety of infections. In postmortem examinations, some AIDS patients have been found to be infected with a staggering variety of bacteria, protozoa, fungi, and viruses. Researchers have faced the difficult task of determining which of these pathogens are merely opportunistic—secondary to the disease state—and which may have caused the disease itself.

Among a significant proportion of AIDS patients, for example, viral studies found an abnormally high number of latent viruses, including cytomegalovirus (CMV), herpes simplex virus, Epstein-Barr virus (EBV), and human T cell leukemia virus (HTLV) among others. Initially, research focused on a possible link between AIDS and CMV, a virus known to cause transient immunosuppression during infection. CMV was for a time the most commonly identified virus in blood samples from AIDS patients. But the results of other studies suggested that CMV was more likely to be an opportunistic agent than the cause of AIDS.

The evidence that linked human T cell leukemia virus to AIDS was strong, but equally ambiguous. HTLV is an example of a retrovirus—a group of viruses known to cause tumors in a number of animals, and suspected of causing certain types of human leukemias. In early studies, approximately 25 percent of AIDS patients showed evidence of the presence of human T cell leukemia virus, compared to only 1 percent of the normal population. HTLV is known to target T cells, the cells that most likely come under attack in AIDS, making it a candidate for a causative agent. But other evidence seemed to argue just as strongly against a role for HTLV in AIDS. HTLV does not kill infected T cells; it transforms them into uncontrollably proliferating cancer cells. Yet AIDS patients show a *decreased* number of helper T cells. If HTLV were indeed the cause, investigators would expect to see T cell tumors in AIDS patients. And yet no cases of such tumors had been reported in the patient population.

Still, while researchers puzzled over this seeming contradiction, new clues continued to point to a link between some form of HTLV virus and AIDS. Not long after the discovery of Acquired Immune Deficiency Syndrome, researchers at the New England Primate Research Center in Massachusetts began to notice an unusually large number of deaths among the center's colony of macaque monkeys. Many of the monkeys had developed lymphomas, immune cell tumors. But the majority of the deaths among the animals resulted from *Candida albicans* and cytomegalovirus infections—some of the same kinds of opportunistic infections being diagnosed in patients with AIDS. Tests of the diseased monkeys confirmed that they were suffering from a number of immunologic abnormalities.

During the same period, a similar outbreak of a mysterious disease occurred at the University of California Primate Research Center in Davis, where twenty-seven monkeys in one cage developed swollen lymph glands, diarrhea, fever, weight loss, and a rare skin cancer. Within eighteen months, all the animals were dead, victims of a wide range of severe infections.

To their surprise, scientists had uncovered a naturally occurring animal model for AIDS.

The scientific team at the New England Primate Research Center began a series of experiments to identify the disease agent. They removed a lymphoma from one monkey and treated it to destroy all the cells in the tumor. The extract was then injected into several healthy animals. Within a short time, several of the animals developed the same type of tumor that was used to prepare the cell-free extract. A number of other animals developed symptoms of the AIDS-like syndrome. The evidence indicated that a virus in the cell-free extract from the tumors had transmitted the disease. In subsequent experiments at the California Primate Center and the National Institutes of Health, investigators found that the AIDS-like disease in monkeys could also be transmitted from diseased rhesus monkeys to healthy monkeys with filtered plasma. And within the first three months of 1984, investigators at the New England and California primate centers reported that they had isolated a virus—a retrovirus in the same family as human T cell leukemia virus—that could produce the AIDS-like disease in healthy rhesus monkeys. The simian retrovirus was isolated from the blood and tissues of diseased macaque and rhesus monkeys and then grown in culture dishes. Within two to four weeks after a group of healthy monkeys was injected with these retrovirus-infected cells, they began to exhibit the full spectrum of disease symptoms associated with the simian form of AIDS.

The evidence strongly suggested that some form of HTLV or related retrovirus was responsible for simian AIDS. And during the same period, studies at the National Cancer Institute were beginning to turn up new evidence that some form of HTLV was also responsible for human AIDS. Research teams under the direction of Robert C. Gallo were beginning to discover the presence of a new form of HTLV (termed HTLV-3) in a significant number of AIDS patients. In a group of 21 patients with symptoms that frequently precede the development of AIDS, for example, 18 were found to have HTLV-3. The virus was also found in 26 of 72 study patients with AIDS, and 3 out of 4 clinically normal women with children who had developed the disease. No evidence of HTLV-3, however, was found in a control study of 115 healthy heterosexual individuals. In a related study, 89 percent of blood samples from AIDS patients showed the presence of antibodies that targeted antigens of HTLV-3, compared to less than 1 percent of healthy heterosexual subjects. The NCI findings, published May 4, 1984 in *Science,* also included the announcement that researchers had developed a laboratory technique for producing HTLV-3 in large quantities, making possible further studies into the nature and behavior of the virus.

Ironically, those studies may prove that HTLV-3 was first discovered not by NCI researchers but by investigators at the Pasteur Institute in Paris, almost a year before. In a paper published May 3, 1983 in *Science,* researchers under the direction of Dr. Luc Montagnier announced the discovery of a previously unknown retrovirus present in a significant number of AIDS patients. The French researchers argued that this new virus, termed Lyphadenopathy-Associated Virus (LAV), was the likely cause of AIDS. Many researchers now suspect that HTLV-3 and LAV are indeed the same virus, one that some investigators have already begun to call HTLV-3/LAV. Studies currently underway are expected to confirm this hypothesis.

Both the French and American findings are supported by several dramatic observations made in March 1984 by Samuel Broder and his colleagues at the National Cancer Institute. The researchers began by generating killer T cells that specifically targeted cells infected with the human T cell leukemia virus. At first these killer T cells were extremely effective in destroying the HTLV-infected cells. But over time they began to lose their ability to kill; inexplicably, the killer T cells stopped growing and eventually died. And when researchers examined the ineffective killer T cells, they made another unexpected discovery: the T cells themselves were now infected with the virus. Somehow the role of killer and victim had become reversed. According to one hypothesis, human T cell leukemia virus may be able to disrupt the normal ability of killer T cells to respond to HTLV antigens on infected cells. Instead of being activated by the presence of these antigens, the killer T cells become inactivated, shutting off their immune responses and eventually dying.

These latest findings offer substantial evidence that HTLV-3/ LAV will prove to be the cause of AIDS. Final proof will come only when researchers are able to infect healthy laboratory animals with the virus and then observe the onset of AIDS-like symptoms. Confirmation may prove difficult, however; only certain animals may be susceptible to the human virus, and its behavior may differ in animals and humans. As this book goes to press, AIDS has yet to be observed in animals inoculated with HTLV-3. Still, most researchers remain confident that subsequent experiments will prove conclusively that HTLV-3/LAV is indeed the cause of the disease. If so, a technique already developed by researchers at the NCI for identifying the presence of HTLV-3 may offer a reliable blood test for the disease. Such a test would allow for the early diagnosis of patients with AIDS, as well as a means to prevent the transmission of AIDS through transfused blood. By identifying the causative agent of the disease, scientists will also have taken the first step necessary in developing a vaccine against AIDS. Most investigators recognize that the preparation of a vaccine may be a long, difficult process, however; indeed, there are still many viral diseases for which effective vaccines have not been achieved.

While researchers in the lab have worked to isolate the cause of AIDS, physicians throughout the world have struggled desperately to treat patients with the disease. No effective way has yet been found to restore immune responsiveness in these patients. Helpless to reverse the severe immunosuppression of the disease, physicians have focused instead on treating the secondary life-threatening infections which are, in effect, only the symptoms of AIDS. Conventional antibiotic, antifungal, and antiprotozoal drugs have been used with some success. But these drugs do not treat the generalized immunosuppression of AIDS, and with virtually no defenses, AIDS patients often go on to develop the same or new infections. In certain cases, reinfections may become increasingly difficult to treat—especially when available drugs have serious side effects. Few patients have been able to survive a third infection of *Pneumocystis* pneumonia, the leading cause of death among AIDS patients.

The struggle to treat Kaposi's sarcoma has been almost as frustrating. At first physicians treated the rare skin cancer with traditional chemotherapies. In certain cases, these drugs reduced the number or size of the skin lesions, but they had one profoundly serious side effect. By attacking immune cells as well as cancer cells, the drugs further suppressed immune functions in patients whose immune systems were already devastated by the disease itself. In the search for a more acceptable treatment, some physicians began to test the lymphokine whose anticancer effects had created such widespread hope: interferon. Preliminary studies have found that alpha and beta interferon may be useful therapeutic agents for controlling Kaposi's sarcoma in a certain number of individuals. But interferon's potential value is limited. It may be helpful in treating Kaposi's sarcoma, but only in rare cases of AIDS is the cancer itself life-threatening. Usually patients succumb to other opportunistic infections. Because interferon can only partially restore some immune functions, even successful interferon treatment leaves AIDS patients susceptible to a variety of potentially lethal infections.

Still, many immunologists believe that interferon, along with other lymphokines, may yet hold out the ultimate hope of treatment for people with AIDS. AIDS patients exhibit profound destruction of the T cell population—the source of several important lymphokines, including interleukin 2 and interferon. Precursor T cells find themselves in an internal environment that lacks the very substances that are essential for their growth and development into functional helper and killer T cells; phagocytes lack the lymphokine signals they need to function effectively; B cells are left without crucial antibody-manufacturing signals.

One lymphokine in particular, interleukin 2, is centrally important to all these immune functions. A number of researchers have wondered whether this potent lymphokine, administered therapeutically, might be able to restore normal immune responses in AIDS patients. The initial laboratory studies of interleukin 2 were promising. Injected into cultures of immune cells from AIDS patients, the lymphokine appeared to restore, at least partially, the activity of killer T cells. Based on these findings, the National Institutes of Health authorized funds to purchase interleukin 2 for preliminary studies with AIDS patients. And in April 1984, tests of interleukin 2 in AIDS patients began in Maryland and California.

Some investigators remain doubtful that interleukin 2 alone will be able to fully restore immune response in vivo, however. As Dr. Gerald V. Quinnan of the Food and Drug Administration has cautioned, "What has been demonstrated is that interleukin 2 can restore the ability of lymphocytes from AIDS patients to kill virus-infected cells in the test tube. But this is a long way from showing the same result can be achieved clinically."* Interleukin 2 is only one of several important lymphokines produced by helper T cells. In AIDS patients, the production of these other, less well understood lymphokines may also be severely disrupted. Unfortunately, many of these substances are not yet available in a pure form. Even basic research into the nature and function of some of them is still in its infancy. Interleukin 2 alone may have some therapeutic value, but it cannot substitute for all the lymphokines produced by normal T cells. The ultimate cure for AIDS may have to await the characterization and purification of the entire range of T cell-derived lymphokines missing in AIDS patients. Then immunologists may be able to prepare a carefully measured combination of the range of different lymphokines produced by healthy T cells. Such a combination could effectively restore the full range of immune functions.

Over the last four years, the clinical treatment of Acquired Immune Deficiency Syndrome and the basic research into the functioning of immune responses have been intimately related. Every new laboratory discovery has been seized by immunologists and fitted into the puzzle of AIDS in the hope of finding both its cause and cure. In the study of AIDS, perhaps more dramatically than in any other disease syndrome, we have discovered that the distance between the knowledge of how immune cells communicate with each other and the successful

---

*Quoted in Marwick, C. 1983. Medical News: Interleukin 2 trial will try to spark flagging immunity of AIDS patients. *JAMA* 250:1125.

treatment of many life-threatening diseases may involve only one step.

seven

THE PARADOX OF REJECTION

Not only in his thoughts, his feelings, and his will, but in the chemical markings of his body each human individual is unlike any other that has ever existed.

SALVADOR E. LURIA, 1973

In many ways, our efforts at protecting and healing the body seem insignificant beside the power and vigilance of the body's own mechanisms of defense. Many of the greatest advances in medical science are nothing more than ways we have discovered to assist or control the healthy functioning of the immune system. Vaccines simply trigger immune responses so that the mechanisms of defense and immunity will protect the body from subsequent attack. Antibiotics, which interrupt the normal life cycle of bacteria and other microbial pathogens by blocking their ability to synthesize RNA, DNA, and proteins, only help to give the immune system a head start in defeating the enemy. Nowhere is the critical importance of a functioning immune system clearer than in our frustrating powerlessness to treat many of the infections that follow the breakdown of normal immune responses in Acquired Immune Deficiency Syndrome.

But there is one situation in which the physician and the immune system become adversaries—when a surgeon may stand by helplessly as he watches the immune system systematically destroy his best efforts at preserving life. We have achieved the ability to lift a human heart from the body of a donor and transplant it, intact and alive, into another human body. Triggered by new nerve impulses, that heart will begin beating—a new, healthy heart to replace a damaged or diseased one. Gradually the organ will grow healthier and stronger—but only for a time. Almost as soon as an organ is transplanted, very small pieces of its tissue are shed into the bloodstream. Some of these fragments make their way to a nearby lymph node, where T cells recognize the grafted tissue's foreign antigens. At the same time, T cells in the blood make direct contact with the graft itself. Activated, these host T cells begin to release migration inhibitory factor, interleukin 2, chemotactic factors, and gamma interferon, recruiting and activating phagocytes, killer T cells and natural killer cells, which swarm toward the graft and begin to attack the foreign cells of the new organ. Unless physicians halt the destructive immune response, the tissues of the graft will begin to hemorrhage and die. The heart, succumbing to the attack, begins to beat irregularly and then not at all. Within several weeks, the process of rejection is complete.

The history of surgical transplantation has been a fierce battle between physician and the host immune system for the survival of the graft—and the life of the patient. In 1954, helplessly watching a 24-year-old man die of chronic kidney disease, doctors at Boston's Peter Bent Brigham Hospital decided to take a desperate chance. Earlier attempts at kidney transplantation had always ended in failure after the massive rejection of the transplanted organ. But this time the surgeons had a powerful advantage. The patient's identical twin brother had agreed to donate a kidney. Because the antigens that determine self are identical in identical twins, the recipient's immune system would accept the grafted tissue as if it were his own. For the first time in medical history, a human organ was successfully transplanted.

Probably the most famous of all transplant operations occurred in 1967, when Dr. Christiaan Barnard performed the first successful heart transplant in Cape Town, South Africa. Since that time, more than five hundred such transplants have been undertaken. Although the surgical techniques are relatively simple, the risk of rejection has been formidable. During the first four years of experiments with the procedure, heart transplant patients rarely lived more than several months after the surgery. Indeed, the survival rate was so discouraging that, for a time, heart transplantation was virtually abandoned.

Rejection has also been the principle obstacle to the transplantation of bone marrow. More than two thousand bone marrow transplants have been performed since Dr. Georges Mathé of the Gustave Roussy Institute near Paris pioneered the procedure in 1963. Bone marrow transplants offer great promise for the treatment of many diseases, including anemia, immunodeficiency syndromes, and even leukemia. But they pose their own special and substantial problem of rejection. Like Mathé's revolutionary surgery, the fundamental goal of all bone marrow transplants is to restore or replace the recipient's bone marrow with a new source of healthy cells, called stem cells, which will then produce the red blood cells, lymphocytes, phagocytes, and other blood cells needed for survival.

But grafted bone marrow also contains small but significant populations of healthy, active T cells. Like the forces hidden within the Trojan horse, these powerful cells, carried behind enemy lines during the transplant procedure, can swiftly bring about the destruction not of the graft, but of the host itself. Transplanted T cells behave like all T cells: they respond to the presence of foreign antigens by attacking and destroying foreign cells. Transplanted T cells find themselves in the midst of an extremely large graft—the entire body of the recipient. Immediately they begin to trigger a series of reactions that severely damage host tissue. And because the recipient's body is usually severely immunosuppressed, either by disease or by the drugs that must be administered to facilitate the graft, transplanted T cells encounter almost no resistance. The disease that results is called *graft versus host disease.* The skin, liver, and gastrointestinal tract are prime targets of graft versus host attack. Within six weeks after a bone marrow transplant, a painful rash may appear as the skin comes under immune attack. The response then spreads to the tissues of the intestines and the blood vessels leaving the liver. In severe cases, graft versus host responses can actually threaten the life of the bone marrow transplant recipient.

Rejection may seem paradoxical—an act of defense which in the end may indirectly kill the body. But there is nothing surprising about the rejection of a transplanted organ. The immune system is simply playing by its own fundamental and absolute rule: the destruction of all foreign cells and substances that invade the body. Over millions of years of evolution the immune system has evolved for this single purpose: to defend the self against invasion from the external environment, from anything that it recognizes as non-self. An attack on transplanted tissue is no different than the attack against an invading pathogen. Indeed, while a first skin graft will be rejected within ten to fourteen days, a second graft from the same donor will be rejected within only two to four days—following precisely the pattern that Robert Koch discovered in his experiments with the tuberculosis pathogen. Memory T cells, present in large numbers after the body's response to the first skin graft, swiftly and vigorously reject the second graft as they would a returning virus or bacterium. Foreign is foreign, and foreign cells must be rejected at all cost—even if the cost of rejection means the death of the host. The immune system cannot deliberate. Without intervention by extraordinary means, rejection follows the overwhelming number of attempts at transplanting tissues or organs.

Still, there are exceptions to the rule—circumstances in which transplanted tissue grows and prospers without triggering rejection. At the turn of the century, cancer biologists first observed these perplexing exceptions; and it is with their experiments that the story of research into the immunologic mechanisms of rejection begins.

Searching for a way to keep individual tumors alive for long-term study, researchers tried to transplant growing tumor cells from one laboratory mouse to another. But virtually every attempt met with failure. The transplanted tumors were almost inevitably rejected by the recipient mice. In rare cases, however, a transplanted tumor would survive and grow in the new host—an exception to the rule. And yet when the surviving tumor was again transplanted into a new mouse, it was almost invariably rejected. There appeared to be no pattern to acceptance or rejection, no way to explain why, while most tumors were swiftly rejected, some seemed to survive.

Then, in 1903, a Danish investigator named Carl Jensen stumbled upon the first glimmerings of an explanation. Jensen was experimenting with an inbred strain of mice that shared closely related or identical genes, the segments of DNA that control everything from hair color to body size. When he isolated a lung tumor from one of the mice and injected it into several other mice of the same strain, he was startled to find that the tumors survived and grew in *all* the recipient mice. The rejection process had not taken place at all. But when Jensen injected the tumor into other, genetically unrelated mice, the tumor was swiftly rejected.

These experiments contained the seeds of a revolutionary idea: tumor rejection, and perhaps the rejection of any type of transplant, had something to do with the genetic makeup of the donor and recipient. The tumor of an inbred mouse, injected into other mice of the same genetic strain, survived and grew. Injected into genetically unrelated mice, however, the same tumor was swiftly destroyed.

In the years that followed, other researchers confirmed Jensen's startling findings. By 1916, most scientists were convinced that a small number of specific genes controlled the acceptance or rejection of foreign transplants. But how genes exerted their control remained uncertain until an English researcher named Peter Gorer discovered the link between certain genes and the mechanisms of graft rejection. In his experiments, Gorer injected a tumor from one albino mouse into another genetically identical albino mouse. And like Jensen before him, he observed that the tumor was accepted by the inbred mouse. He repeated the experiment, this time injecting the albino mouse tumor into two unrelated strains, agouti and black mice. As Gorer had expected, the tumor was swiftly rejected by the genetically unrelated black mouse. But to his considerable surprise, the tumor was *not* rejected by the agouti mouse. Indeed, the tumor survived and grew just as it would if the donor and recipient had been genetically identical. And yet the albino and agouti were genetically unrelated strains. Why had the tumor survived?

From previous experiments Gorer knew that albino and agouti mice were, in most ways, very different in their genetic makeup; but he had found that they did share a common form of one antigen on the surface of their cells—an antigen Gorer called antigen II. The strain of black mice lacked this specific form of antigen II. By crossbreeding the three strains, Gorer discovered that any mouse that possessed the albino mouse form of antigen II on its cells would accept the albino tumor; mice that lacked this specific surface protein would reject the tumor.

Gorer had made a monumental discovery: the presence or absence of a specific form of antigen II on the recipient's cells appeared to determine whether the albino tumor was accepted or rejected by the immune system. Later experiments revealed that what Gorer had called antigen II actually consisted of several related antigens, which came to be called *histocompatibility antigens.* Like all antigens, histocompatibility antigens are nothing more than proteins that appear on the surface of cells. What sets histocompatibility antigens apart is the force of the immune responses they generate when they are detected by a foreign host. These antigens, which appear in unique forms on the surface of virtually all cells, are the major antigenic stimulus for rejection. Large numbers of T cells are programmed to identify histocompatibility antigens. If they encounter antigens identical to those found on the body's own cells, they make no response, and the transplant will be accepted. But if T cells detect a foreign form of histocompatibility antigen, they respond swiftly against the cells that bear it.

The discovery of histocompatibility antigens in laboratory mice initiated an intensive search for a similar set of antigens in humans. And in the late 1950s, the search at last turned up the presence of unique histocompatibility antigens on human cells. These antigens, discovered first on human white blood cells, are called *human leukocyte antigens,* or *HLA antigens.* They are the human counterparts of the mouse histocompatibility antigens, and like them, HLA antigens play a pivotal role in the acceptance or rejection of all types of human transplants. Transplants between identical twins, who share identical HLA antigens, are almost always accepted. But transplants between genetically nonidentical individuals, even between parents and their children, are usually rejected because of the differences in the pattern of HLA antigens. The HLA antigens are like cellular fingerprints. They mark the cells within our bodies as self. When those cells are transplanted to a new body during the grafting of tissue or organ, these same antigens signal the presence of non-self—the enemy—and rejection begins.

The rejection of a transplanted organ or tissue, triggered by histocompatibility antigens, is cell-mediated—carried out by killer T cells and phagocytes in direct cell-to-cell combat. Another form of transplant, the transfusion of blood from one individual to another, can trigger a very different form of rejection, mediated by antibodies. The antigens that mark red blood cells are distinct from histocompatibility antigens. They were first identified by the German immunologist Karl Landsteiner in 1901. He found that human red blood cells bear unique surface antigens, which he called *A-antigen* and *B-antigen.* When Landsteiner tested blood from various individuals, he recognized four possible configurations of these antigens. Some people had only A-antigens on their red blood cells, while others had only B-antigens. A small number of people had red blood cells that bore both A- and B-antigens, while others had red blood cells that bore neither antigen. Landsteiner described these four blood types as A, B, AB, and O—a classification that remains in effect today. (In the United States, approximately 45 percent of the population is type O, 42 percent type A, 10 percent type B, and 3 percent type AB.)

In subsequent experiments, Landsteiner observed an interesting property of blood cells that bear different antigens. When he mixed whole blood from a type A individual with serum (the fluid part of blood, containing no blood cells) from a type B individual, the type A red cells quickly formed very large clumps, visible to the naked eye. He repeated the experiment, this time mixing type B blood with serum from a type A individual. The type B red cells formed large clumps. These clumps did not form, however, when Landsteiner mixed blood cells and serum from the same individual, or when he mixed blood cells and serum from two different individuals with the same blood type. Landsteiner's observations suggested that some factor in the serum of an individual with one blood type was making the red blood cells of an individual with a different blood type clump together.

That factor, he later discovered, was antibody. Individuals with type A blood appeared to have circulating antibodies against the B-antigen that was *absent* from their own red blood cells. Blood type B individuals had antibodies against the A-antigen they lacked. Type AB individuals, who had both A- and B-antigens on their red blood cells, had no circulating antibodies against either antigen. And type O individuals, whose blood cells carried neither antigen, had circulating antibodies against both A-antigens and B-antigens. When certain types of antigenically different blood samples were mixed, the antibodies from one sample would bind to the antigens they recognized on the red blood cells from the other sample. Antibodies have two sites for binding antigens—the two arms of the Y-shaped antibody molecule. In the clumping reaction, one antibody arm binds the A- or B-antigen on one cell and the other arm binds the identical antigen on a second cell. Large numbers of these antigen-antibody bonds cause the visible clumping of red blood cells.

Landsteiner's discoveries helped explain the severe reactions of fever and anemia that sometimes occur when blood is transfused from one individual to another. When a type A individual receives type B blood containing antibodies against the A-antigen, for example, these antibodies quickly bind to the A-antigen on the recipient's red cells. Antibody attracts complement proteins, which gather on the red blood cell membrane and set in motion the destruction of the cell. Since Landsteiner's discovery of A- and B-antigens, researchers have identified over three hundred additional blood group antigens. Fortunately, only a small number of these antigens can trigger a severe transfusion reaction when donor and recipient are mismatched. Current clinical practices involve typing donor and recipient for antigens of the ABO system and one other major blood group antigen, called RhD. Blood typing refers to Rh positive or Rh negative, depending on whether or not red blood cells bear the unique RhD antigen. By matching both ABO and RhD antigens, physicians can avoid an adverse reaction to transfusion.

The nature of histocompatibility antigens, however, is far more complex, and the problems of rejection of tissue and organ transplants have been correspondingly difficult. Only in the last three decades has the idea of replacing a diseased organ with a new, healthy one moved from the realm of dreams to clinical reality; and even now, the precision and sophistication of new surgical techniques have far outpaced our ability to control the host immune system in order to prevent rejection.

The conventional weapon against rejection has been the use of drugs and radiation therapies that suppress the immune system by blocking the growth of immune cells. Unfortunately, the drugs we have had available—drugs like Cytoxan, Imuran, and steroids—block the synthesis of DNA in all dividing cells, effectively killing not only the cells involved in rejection, but the full arsenal of immune cells, as well as other dividing cells in the body. In fact, many of the drugs used to control rejection are also used in cancer therapy in an effort to destroy tumor cells. By blocking the growth of immune cells, conventional chemotherapy leaves the body seriously compromised in its ability to fight invading bacteria, viruses, and other pathogens. And by blocking the growth of other cells in the body, these drugs produce an array of serious side effects. For physicians, the use of immunosuppressive drugs and radiation has created a kind of "Catch-22." If a transplant is to survive, they must severely suppress the patient's immune system; but immunosuppression exposes the patient to the dangerous risk of developing potentially lethal infections.

One way to reduce the potential for rejection, and the need for severe immunosuppression, is to select donors and recipients whose histocompatibility antigens are similar. In the past, physicians have looked for donors among family members. Identical twins possess identical histocompatibility antigens, and there is virtually no risk of rejection. Among siblings, the chances of finding shared histocompatibility antigens is about one in four. But when genetically similar family members are not available, transplant patients must turn to unrelated individuals, and the chance of finding a good match is less than one in a thousand.

By learning more about the range of histocompatibility antigens, however, immunologists have begun to find ways to measure the histocompatibility similarities between unrelated individuals and better the chances of finding a good match. In one matching technique, blood samples from donor and recipient are exposed to a series of antibodies that target known histocompatibility antigens. Complement proteins are then added to the blood. When an antibody specific for a certain histocompatibility antigen binds in the presence of complement to lymphocytes in the blood samples, the destruction of these cells indicates the presence of that specific antigen on the cell membrane. Researchers can then compare the effects of different antibodies on the two blood samples and measure the degree of histocompatibility differences.

Unfortunately, histocompatibility typing is a long, expensive process, and not always successful. Immunologists have identified and learned to test for some seventy histocompatibility antigens; but there are important ones that have yet to be identified. And researchers have found other factors that can influence the fate of grafted tissue. Female-to-male transplants, for example, may be rejected even when a good histocompatibility match is made—the result, some researchers believe, of a histocompatibility factor associated with the male Y chromosome. Still, each histocompatibility match between donor and recipient increases the chance of a successful transplant, and matching has become a crucial feature of successful transplant therapy.

The greatest spur to transplant surgery in the last several years, however, has come with the unexpected discovery, in 1970, of a revolutionary new drug called *cyclosporin A.* While investigating soil samples gathered from Wisconsin and Norway, researcher Jean Borel of the Swiss pharmaceutical company Sandoz discovered two kinds of fungus that produced a substance with an unprecedented power. Injected into a culture of lymphocytes, the substance, called cyclosporin A, somehow blocked the ability of the immune cells to grow or function; but unlike any other immunosuppressive drugs, cyclosporin A did not appear to kill the lymphocytes. At first it was thought that the drug interfered with the ability of interleukin 2 to stimulate the growth and development of T cells. But experiments demonstrated that cyclosporin A actually blocked the ability of interleukin 1 to induce the production of interleukin 2. Without interleukin 2, T cells could neither divide nor carry on their activities as helper or killer T cells. By targeting a crucial link in the lymphokine cycle, cyclosporin A effectively sabotaged a wide range of important immune responses.

Cyclosporin A promised to be nothing short of a wonder

drug for transplant surgery. The specificity of its effect would give it a crucial advantage over conventional immunosuppressive drugs. Cyclosporin A could block the function of immune cells while it left other cells in the body undisturbed, eliminating many of the severe toxic side effects which accompanied other drugs, and which often left patients seriously debilitated. In 1977, Dr. David J. G. White of Cambridge University and Dr. Roy Y. Calne of Addenbrooke's Hospital in Cambridge began the first tests of cyclosporin A in experimental organ transplants with laboratory animals. The new drug quickly fulfilled its promise, significantly increasing the survival of transplanted hearts and kidneys. In the following years it was used for the first time in human kidney and heart transplant patients. And in 1983, after tests with more than two thousand such patients in the United States, cyclosporin A was approved by the Food and Drug Administration.

Already the drug has brought about a revolution in transplant surgery. Kidney transplants, which had only a 50 percent chance of surviving the first year with conventional immunosuppressive drug therapy, now have more than an 80 percent chance of survival with cyclosporin A. The success rate for liver transplants has doubled, from 35 percent to 70 percent. Cyclosporin A has also shown great promise in the prevention of graft versus host disease in bone marrow recipients. In the future, as physicians learn precisely how best to administer cyclosporin A, the chances of success in many different kinds of transplant surgery will no doubt improve even more.

Cyclosporin A has dramatically reduced the risk of rejection in transplant surgery; but its effect is still to block the full range of normal immune responses, and patients on the drug still run a serious risk of severe infection. To be fully safe and effective, the ideal transplant therapy would target only those immune responses directed against the histocompatibility antigens of the graft itself, leaving other immune cells free to fight infection. In essence, the ideal transplant therapy would produce a state of highly specific immune tolerance to the graft, tricking the body into accepting non-self antigens as self. Unfortunately, the ideal immunosuppressive drug does not yet exist. But several provocative experiments have suggested what form such a therapy might take.

In the late 1950s, researchers R. E. Billingham, L. Brent, and Sir Peter Medawar discovered an extraordinary technique —a way to trick the immune system of a laboratory mouse into accepting a foreign skin graft. They injected fetal and newborn white mice with cells from brown mice—two strains with very different histocompatibility antigens. When the white mice reached adulthood, the researchers transplanted skin grafts from the brown mice to the mature white mice. Under normal circumstances, because of the histocompatibility differences between the two strains, the skin grafts would have been rejected within two weeks. Instead, these grafts were readily and completely accepted by the white mice. Somehow, the injection of cells from brown mice into neonatal white mice had created a state of tolerance in the white mice that allowed the acceptance of a foreign skin graft as if it were self.

The experiments of Billingham, Brent, and Medawar were a major turning point in transplantation research. They demonstrated for the first time that it was possible to circumvent the barrier of histocompatibility antigens in tissue transplants—in a sense, to change non-self into self. Unfortunately, the induction of stable, long-term tolerance in adult animals has proved far more difficult, indicating that tolerance to self antigens develops very early in life. Still, their findings have led researchers to a related approach to preventing transplant rejection, one that may soon prove useful in human patients.

In one series of experiments that spanned twelve years, Brent and his colleagues at St. Mary's Hospital Medical School in London constructed an extremely effective procedure for the prevention of skin graft rejection in adult laboratory mice. The key to their success was the merging of several empirical techniques, each of which was already known to induce a partial state of tolerance to foreign antigens. Researchers had discovered that by injecting donor antigens directly into the bloodstream (a route by which the body rarely encounters antigens) they could sometimes induce a state of tolerance rather than immunity in the prospective recipient. How the injection of antigens creates a state of temporary tolerance is still not well understood. But Brent and his colleagues later uncovered at least one of the immunologic mechanisms that appear to be at work. They began their experiment by preparing an extract of liver cells from a donor mouse and injecting the extract intravenously into other mice. Sixteen days later, skin grafts were taken from the same donor and transplanted to the prepared mice. To better the chances of acceptance, the researchers also injected the grafted animals with serum that contained antibodies against lymphocytes. These antilymphocyte antibodies would reduce the number of T cells capable of attacking and rejecting the graft.

The results were dramatic. In untreated control animals, all grafted tissue was quickly rejected. But in the treated animals, as many as 50 percent of the grafts were accepted. By adding the limited use of procarbazine, a powerful immunosuppressive drug, to the protocol, the investigators were able to achieve an impressive 85 percent rate of survival for grafted tissue. Through some unknown mechanism, they discovered, the combination of a prior exposure to donor antigens and the administration of antilymphocyte antibodies and procarbazine induces in the mice the production of suppressor T cells that selectively block only those immune responses directed against the specific foreign skin graft. When the researchers tried to graft other tissue from unrelated mice, the grafts were vigorously rejected.

Although much research remains to be done, this protocol offers exciting potential for transplant therapy. Ironically, one element of the procedure may already be in clinical practice. A number of kidney transplant centers have begun to give recipients transfusions of donor blood prior to the kidney transplant because they have been found to increase the chances that the graft will be accepted. Many researchers now believe that the transfusions may induce the production of suppressor cells that specifically prevent rejection responses directed against the transplanted organ.

In the future, perhaps, we may develop far more direct ways to control the power of suppressor cells to inhibit or halt immune responses directed at specific histocompatibility antigens. Evidence suggests that suppressor T cells may issue their commands in the language of lymphokines. If we can learn to produce these suppressor lymphokines, we may be able to use them to prevent immune responses against specific foreign tissue. Indeed, it may someday be possible to prepare a panel of suppressor lymphokines, each of which would block immune responses against a specific histocompatibility antigen.

Most of the efforts of transplant immunologists have been directed at this one goal: finding a fully effective way to circumvent the immune system's deliberate and absolute destruction of any cell or substance that bears foreign antigens. The potential use of immunosuppressive lymphokines, like Brent's three-part protocol, is nothing more, really, than a way to trick the immune system into making one exception to its most fundamental rule: the destruction of anything that is non-self.

Curiously, there already exists in nature a profound exception to the fundamental rule of defense—one case in which the body permits foreign cells to grow and prosper. It is an exception on which the continuation of most life depends.

eight

OLD MEETS NEW

Everything in a living being is centered on reproduction.

FRANÇOIS JACOB, 1973

Each new human life begins with the joining of sperm and egg, and in that moment an extraordinarily complex process begins. For scientists in many fields of research, there is much that remains mysterious about the process of conception and gestation. For immunologists, the greatest mystery is that it takes place at all.

The fundamental rule of the immune system—the swift and unequivocal rejection of cells and substances bearing foreign antigens—would seem to make the joining of sperm and egg and the growth of a fetus impossible. Sperm cells are strongly antigenic. They carry on their cell membranes a variety of HLA antigens (the most important antigens involved in graft rejection) as well as ABO blood group antigens, all of them extremely powerful in triggering immune responses. In theory, at least, sperm cells introduced into the female reproductive tract should be detected as foreign and destroyed. Repeated coitus between two sexual partners should, in fact, result in the female's complete immunity to the male's sperm cells. According to the rules of immune response, repeated coitus is no different from the process of vaccination. The first time foreign sperm cells "invade," the female body, responding to their foreign antigens, should trigger the production of long-lived memory T and B cells. Upon any subsequent exposure to the same antigens, these memory cells should then respond by swiftly destroying the cells that bear them. (An egg that did manage to become impregnated, and which from that moment bears antigens foreign to the mother's body, should itself be swiftly destroyed.)

Of course this does not happen, except in the rarest cases; and the provocative question for immunologists is why it does not.

Research into the immunologic strategies that protect sperm cells from attack have uncovered some astonishing answers. Sperm leave the male reproductive system coated with protective substances derived in part from seminal fluid. To determine the role these substances might play in protecting sperm, researchers "washed" the sperm cells of laboratory animals, removing their protective covering. When these cells were then introduced into the female reproductive tract, they immediately triggered the production of antisperm antibodies—demonstrating decisively the protective role these substances play.

Many researchers believe that the covering of seminal fluid

substances may allow sperm cells to hide their antigens, thus eluding detection by the female immune system. Specific molecules in seminal fluid also appear to have the power to block the development of a potentially lethal attack by complement proteins. And there is even some evidence that seminal fluid contains substances that may actually be able to suppress the activity of T and B cells in the female immune system.

An additional coating of substances which sperm take on within the female reproductive tract may also serve to mask sperm antigens. Because these substances are produced by the female and bear female antigens, they allow sperm cells to make their passage disguised as self. And there may be another way that the female immune system protects sperm cells. Researchers have recently identified the presence of special *nontoxic* antisperm antibodies in the female reproductive tract—antibodies that can bind harmlessly to antigens on the sperm cell that would otherwise become targets of maternal T cells. Binding to sperm cells, nontoxic antibodies also prevent harmful toxic antisperm antibodies that may already exist in the female reproductive tract from binding and destroying them. In this way, the female immune system actually protects sperm from an attack by the female immune system's own cells.

In most cases, the mechanisms sperm cells employ for defense are so powerful that the female immune system simply does not respond to their presence; they make their way completely undetected. There are exceptions, however—cases in which sperm cells fail to elude detection and come under attack by maternal T cells and antibodies—and some researchers have come to believe that the breakdown of normal protective strategies may be among the causes of infertility. Abnormally high levels of antisperm antibodies have been found in the reproductive tracts of a significant number of infertile women —proof that an immune response against sperm cells has taken place. These antisperm antibodies may be able to detect and destroy sperm cells before they are able to reach the egg. Women with unusually high levels of such antibodies have also been found to have a higher rate of miscarriage, which may occur because antisperm antibodies are also able to recognize and target certain structures on the female egg itself. By binding to the egg, antisperm antibodies may prevent it from implanting itself and developing properly in the uterus.

Antisperm antibodies are triggered by the presence of sperm antigens, and their continued production depends on continued exposure to sperm cells. When the sexual partners of women with high antibody levels have initiated the use of condoms during sexual intercourse, effectively eliminating exposure to sperm antigens, researchers have observed a dramatic drop in the level of antisperm antibodies. For some women, this practice has provided an unexpected cure for infertility. More than half of previously infertile women in one study eventually became pregnant after their antisperm antibody levels had been reduced by the use of protective condoms.

Female antibodies may also cause certain types of infertility by targeting components of the female reproductive system itself. Researchers have found a significant number of infertile women with circulating antibodies that target antigens found on the *zona pellucida,* the tissue that surrounds the egg. Such autoantibodies are rarely if ever found in normally fertile women. But in one study of twenty-one infertile women, fifteen had antibodies targeted against their own eggs. Researchers have speculated that these antibodies may coat the surface of the zona pellucida, preventing fertilization or proper implantation of the egg in the uterus.

Male infertility may result, in certain cases, from the attack by the male immune system against its own sperm cells. Because sperm cells develop relatively late in the male, after the body has established tolerance to self antigens, the male immune system does not recognize sperm antigens as self. Male immune cells, coming in contact with sperm, will recognize them as foreign and begin an immune response against them. In most cases, fortunately, sperm cells and the cells of the male immune system never meet. A natural barrier stands between sperm cells and blood, preventing immune cells from detecting and attacking sperm. When this barrier is breached, however, the male immune system will begin to produce autoantibodies directed against sperm. These autoantibodies can bind to sperm cells, blocking their ability to move in a controlled way. (The barrier can be breached during vasectomies, for example, and up to one year after the procedure as many as 70 percent of patients show evidence of circulating autoantibodies.)

Reproductive immunologists are profoundly interested in autoantibodies and their potential role in male infertility. While fewer than 3 percent of fertile men show evidence of antisperm antibodies in their blood, as many as 21 percent of infertile men have been found to have these antibodies. In addition, researchers testing the seminal fluid of infertile men have discovered elevated levels of antisperm IgA—the class of antibody predominant in body secretions. These local autoantibodies, some immunologists believe, may be more significant in male infertility than those circulating in the blood.

By coming to understand the immunologic defects which result in certain kinds of infertility, researchers have also discovered ways to *produce* a state of infertility. In fact, a great deal of research has already gone into the development of an immunologic contraceptive vaccine. The theory behind such a vaccine is relatively simple. Immunologists hope to isolate a specific component of either sperm cells, eggs, or the placenta which will act as a powerful antigenic trigger. By injecting one of these antigens, researchers would be able to immunize a woman against that particular component of the reproductive cycle. The antigen would trigger the production of autoantibodies, which would then bind with the specific component and block contraception or gestation.

But while the idea is simple, the task of developing a contraceptive vaccine has proved to be complex. To be of practical value, a contraceptive vaccine should meet several demanding criteria. The antigen it targets should be specific to the reproductive system, so that the immune response is directed only against the antigen found in reproductive tissues, and not against tissues in other parts of the body. Equally important, the antigen must be specifically involved in conception or gestation, so that a response against it does not affect the timing of or events associated with the menstrual cycle. The immunity generated against the contraceptive antigen should also be reversible, to permit conception at a later time. Finally, it should be possible to produce large quantities of the antigen easily and inexpensively. This is especially important if the contraceptive vaccine is to be of practical value in the birth control programs of poor, underdeveloped countries.

In searching for a suitable antigen, researchers turned first to an antigen found on sperm—a protein called *lactic acid dehydrogenase-X* (LDH-X). In a series of experiments, investigators injected antibodies directed against LDH-X into laboratory animals. The result was a dramatic decrease in fertility. Some of the animals injected with the antibody, however, did become pregnant. That result was not surprising. Ejaculate contains hundreds of millions of sperm cells. To be completely effective, a contraceptive vaccine against sperm antigens would have to contain enough antibody to neutralize every single sperm cell. The total level of LDH-X antigens may have far exceeded the neutralizing capacity of the injected antibodies. Almost any antibody directed against sperm cells could well face the same drawback.

For that reason, investigators have also explored the use of antigens associated with the egg—particularly antigens of the zona pellucida, the coat that surrounds the egg. In theory, an antibody targeted against this coat should bind with the surface cells and thereby prevent sperm cells from penetrating the egg. Even if fertilization were to take place, the antibody would prevent the egg from being successfully implanted in the uterus. In laboratory studies, investigators injected antibodies prepared against antigens of the zona pellucida into test animals, and the result was a significant decrease in fertility. In one series of experiments, 96 percent of the matings by female rats immunized against zona pellucida antigens failed to result in conception. And this state of contraceptive immunity was found to last as long as six months in the laboratory animals.

Normal conception and gestation depend not only on sperm and egg, of course, but on the release of a complex sequence of hormones. Some researchers have wondered if specific antibodies might be used to block the production of a crucial hormone and thus prevent gestation. Studies of one such hormone, a protein called *human chorionic gonadotro-*

phin (HCG), have had encouraging results. HCG is normally produced within six to eight days after fertilization. Its role is to inform the female reproductive system that conception has occurred. The reproductive system then responds by releasing other hormones that set in motion a number of important events that will promote the proper development of the fetus. By injecting antibodies against HCG into laboratory animals, investigators have had significant success in preventing pregnancy. Even more encouraging, the effect of HCG antibodies is reversible. Within a short time after the antibody injections were stopped, the animals conceived. Studies with female volunteers have shown that anti-HCG antibody levels can be maintained for as long as five hundred days without negative side effects or the disruption of the normal menstrual cycle.

There is still a great deal of research and clinical testing to be done before immunologic vaccines become fully safe and effective. But most researchers are confident that this new form of contraception will be available within the next few years.

The life of a sperm cell is very brief, and the passage it must make through enemy territory is a short one. Its defensive strategies must protect it only until it reaches the egg. For the developing fetus, however, the job of defense is far more demanding. From the moment of conception until birth, the fetus is an enemy within the mother's body. A fetus is endowed with the genetic contributions of both parents—genes that will dictate not only hair and eye color, height and weight, and intellectual potential, but also the unique mixture of maternal and paternal antigens that the fetus bears on each of its cells.

Except in very rare circumstances, the fetus will always accept this combination of antigens as self.

But for the mother, each and every cell of the fetus is marked as foreign and targeted for the same destruction that would meet an invading pathogen or surgical transplant. The maternal immune system has the potential to destroy the fetus swiftly and completely. If a paternal skin graft or organ, composed of cells that bear many of the same surface antigens as the developing fetus, is transplanted to the mother, the cells of her immune system will detect it as foreign and swiftly reject it. Even more astonishing: a graft of skin from a newborn infant, transplanted to the mother shortly after she has given birth, will be dead in a matter of days.

Immunologists have uncovered a variety of extraordinary strategies by which the fetus protects itself from attack in the midst of this immunologically hostile environment. These discoveries have given us a new understanding of the complex and paradoxical relationship between mother and fetus—a relationship that is at once nurturing and potentially deadly.

The maternal bloodstream supplies the fetus with the oxygen and nutrients it needs to survive; but the same bloodstream carries a large force of maternal T cells and B cells targeted to attack and destroy the cells of the developing child. Somehow the fetus must be protected from these cells while the nutrients it needs are permitted to pass. This delicate exchange is accomplished across an extremely thin layer of tissue within the placenta. Part of this tissue is supplied by the mother's body and bears her antigens. Another part, called the *trophoblast*, is derived from the fetus, and bears its own unique antigens. Oxygen and nutrients can pass from the mother's blood across the trophoblast into the bloodstream of the fetus, but the blood of mother and fetus do not mix. Only the trophoblast comes in contact with the cells of the mother's immune system. Hence the trophoblast, because it bears antigens foreign to the mother, stands as the first line of defense for the developing child.

The trophoblast is under constant attack by the maternal immune system. Like other cells of the body, the trophoblast bears histocompatibility antigens—the antigens that trigger the powerful mechanisms of graft rejection. And their presence would seem to guarantee the swift destruction of the trophoblast, and with it the fetus. In most instances, the greater the differences in histocompatibility, the greater the potential for a swift and complete rejection. Yet just the opposite appears to be the case in the relationship of mother and fetus. Investigators have found to their surprise that the greater the differences in histocompatibility antigens between mother and father (and thus between mother and fetus), the greater the probability that a *healthy* child will be born. In fact, the size of the placenta and fetus in laboratory mice is directly proportional to the number of differences in histocompatibility genes and antigens between the mother and father. And when investigators have removed lymph nodes nearest the placenta in laboratory animals prior to or during pregnancy, leaving the animals unable to mount a fully effective immune response, the weight of the fetus and placenta have also been found to be significantly lower than normal. These findings seem to contradict everything that immunologists have come to know about the rules of immune response. Indeed, one of the most surprising and perplexing findings in the study of reproductive immunology is that a *strong* maternal immune response against the fetus may actually be essential for its health and proper development.

The reason lies in the special nature of the trophoblast, and the tricks it must play to subvert the maternal immune system and protect the fetus.

The trophoblast bears a unique group of antigens with the formidable name *trophoblast-lymphocyte cross-reactive antigens.* These antigens protect the trophoblast and fetus by triggering the production of a special class of maternal antibodies called *enhancing antibodies.* Enhancing antibodies are functionally identical to the nontoxic antibodies that protect sperm cells on their passage through the female reproductive tract. Unlike most maternal antibodies, enhancing antibodies do not cause the activation of the lethal cascade of complement proteins. Indeed, they are called enhancing antibodies because their role is to enhance the chances that the fetus will survive. By binding to the surface of trophoblast cells, these unique antibodies actually form a protective covering that effectively prevents killer T cells from recognizing and attacking the cells of the trophoblast and fetus. When enhancing antibodies bind to a cell, the antigens that would normally cause an immune response aga against that cell may be withdrawn into the cell, where they disappear from view. In the absence of these antigens, killer T cells of the maternal immune system lack a target for their attack.

Investigators have succeeded in demonstrating the protective power of enhancing antibodies in experiments with skin grafts. In virtually every case, skin grafts on laboratory animals are swiftly and completely rejected. But if the laboratory animals are pregnant and producing enhancing antibodies, a paternal skin graft has a significantly greater chance of survival. Once the animals have given birth and the level of enhancing antibodies drops, however, a paternal skin graft will be swiftly rejected. But as long as high levels of enhancing antibodies are in the bloodstream, paternal grafts are afforded substantial protection from attack—the same protection that defends the fetus during gestation. In fact, enhancing antibodies offer such powerful protection that researchers have even experimented with using them directly to suppress the rejection of grafted tissue or organs in transplant patients.

There is an interesting clinical sidelight to these findings. Researchers have discovered that women who suffer chronic miscarriages may not be producing sufficient amounts of enhancing antibodies to provide the fetus necessary protection against the attack of killer T cells. In a recent study, researchers found that four women with histories of chronic miscarriage all shared an unusually high number of histocompatibility genes and antigens with their husbands. The lack of histocompatibility differences between husband and wife had apparently resulted in a limited maternal immune response against the fetus—including the production of abnormally low quantities of enhancing antibodies. The researchers attempted to generate a strong immune response in these women by injecting blood cells taken from donors with very different histocompatibility types. These antigenically potent cells triggered a full-scale immune response, which included the production of enhancing antibodies. Three of the women in the study went on to give birth to healthy infants.

Researchers have found that toxemia—one of the most serious of all pregnancy-related diseases, and the cause of almost one-third of all maternal deaths in the United States—is far more prevalent among couples exhibiting fewer than normal histocompatibility differences. The exact nature of toxemia remains a mystery, although many clues suggest that it may have an immunologic basis. It is a disease of first pregnancies, rarely occurring in subsequent pregnancies. This suggests that toxemia may result from an abnormal maternal immune response to the foreign antigens of the fetus. After developing toxemia in a first pregnancy, a woman may well develop immunity to those antigens, in much the same way a first exposure to any antigen can create a state of immunity. If a woman who has experienced toxemia conceives a child with a new mate, however, the new form of fetal antigens can pose a renewed threat of toxemia. For the mother, toxemia can result in a steep rise in blood pressure, edema and, in the most serious cases, severe convulsions. For the fetus, the lack of sufficient enhancing antibodies in toxemic women may leave it vulnerable to attack by killer T cells. Researchers have found that women with toxemia often have vascular lesions in the blood vessels of the placenta identical to lesions seen in grafted organs undergoing rejection.

Along with the specialized cross-reactive antigens that trigger enhancing antibodies, the trophoblast bears antigens that target it for attack by the maternal immune system. Curiously, the trophoblast can use even these antigens in self-defense. Under immune attack, the trophoblast can simply shed its antigens into the environment of the womb, where they act as decoy targets for maternal immune cells and antibodies, drawing attention away from the trophoblast and fetus. As more antigens are released and carried in the bloodstream to distant sites, increasingly large numbers of maternal immune cells and antibodies are tied up in chasing decoys. In certain instances, the trophoblast may even shed its own cells, which are carried into the mother's body, where they are eventually destroyed by phagocytes.

The trophoblast does more than simply subvert maternal

antibodies; it can actually enlist these antibodies to protect the fetus. Although many of the antibodies produced by the mother are directed against the antigens of the fetus, other maternal antibodies target pathogens like bacteria and viruses —pathogens to which the fetus is also prey. Because the trophoblast possesses the same cell surface antigens as the fetus itself, the trophoblast can act as a selective filter, binding the antibodies that are directed against the fetus while permitting other helpful antibodies to pass through.

The antibodies that are allowed to reach the fetus can be critically important for its survival—not only during gestation, but after the child is born as well. The maternal antibodies that pass across the trophoblast continue to circulate in the newborn's bloodstream, protecting it against infection for as long as six months after birth, during a period when the infant's own immune system is still developing. Additional maternal antibodies are passed from mother to child during the first months of life. Mother's milk has been found to be rich in antibodies, particularly IgA. Most of these maternal antibodies remain in the infant's gastrointestinal tract, where they provide substantial protection against pathogens that commonly infect that site. In addition, as many as one hundred million active immune cells can be transferred in a single feeding of mother's milk. Incredibly, a breast-fed infant may receive as many T and B cells from its mother each day as are contained in its own body.

Fortunately, these transferred immune cells are not very active against the cells of the newborn child. Most of them, like the maternal antibodies, defend against pathogens of the gastrointestinal tract, specifically targeting organisms to which the infant is particularly vulnerable. For example, 84 percent of cases of infant meningitis are caused by one particular strain of the bacterium *Escherichia coli;* and a high percentage of the maternal T cells in mother's milk specifically target this single strain. Studies have shown that maternal T cells transfer protection against a number of other common gastrointestinal pathogens as well. Thus, mother's milk offers substantial immune protection for the child. And indeed, researchers in the United Kingdom have found that the mortality rate was six times lower in breast-fed infants than in bottle-fed infants.

The production of enhancing antibodies, the shedding of trophoblast antigens, and the selective binding of harmful antibodies all offer substantial protection to the fetus. But they are not fail-safe mechanisms. And the continuation of life is of such overriding importance that the fetus itself has evolved additional defensive measures to help insure its own survival. Researchers have found that the fetus can produce a variety of substances that directly suppress the activity of maternal immune cells, particularly T cells. If the first line of trophoblast defense is breached, the fetus can defend itself by releasing large amounts of immunosuppressive proteins such as alpha-fetoprotein, alpha and beta globulins, or smaller nonprotein immunosuppressive molecules such as progesterone, which will block maternal immune responses against it. Serum from pregnant females added to immune cells in culture dishes will dramatically suppress the immune responses of those cells, because of the presence of immunosuppressive factors produced by the fetus.

And while the fetus suppresses the activity of the mother's helper and killer T cells, it also appears to be able to *generate* the production of maternal suppressor T cells, which selectively turn off maternal immune responses. This devious piece of immunologic trickery is not well understood. But investigators have been able to demonstrate the presence of suppressor T cells in pregnant women that specifically suppress *only* those immune responses targeted against the fetus.

These findings, exciting in their own right, may have far-reaching implications. For immunologists have begun to recognize that breakthroughs in understanding how the fetus manages to survive in the immunologically hostile environment of the female reproductive tract may teach us a great deal about how other foreign cells—specifically cancer cells—survive in the immunologically hostile environment of the body itself.

One of the great debates in immunology and in cancer research has focused on the question of whether or not the immune system can recognize and destroy cancer cells that arise spontaneously in the body. Both immunosuppressed and immunodeficient patients have a significantly higher incidence of certain kinds of tumors—convincing evidence that an active immune surveillance system is normally at work to detect and destroy cancer cells. In some instances, however, the system fails, and these cells are allowed to survive.

Within the last few years, a number of new findings have led researchers to an amazing hypothesis: cancer cells may manage to protect themselves from attack by the immune system in much the same way the trophoblast defends the fetus.

Like trophoblast cells, tumor cells appear to be able to shed decoy antigens and coat themselves with a layer of nontoxic antibodies. The survival of a tumor, like the survival of the fetus, appears to depend on the balance between enhancing antibodies and toxic antibodies. If that balance favors enhancing antibodies, the tumor may be able to survive. If the balance shifts to toxic antibodies, however, the tumor can be destroyed. Immunologists do not yet understand the mechanisms that determine this critical balance. But we do know that tumor cells can secrete certain molecules which severely depress the strength of immune responses against them. Many of the substances released by cancer cells—alpha-fetoprotein, for example—are identical to the molecules released by the fetus to protect itself. And researchers have discovered that tumors produce an immunosuppressive protein smaller and even more powerful than alpha-fetoprotein. Injected into laboratory mice, this protein, simply called immunosuppressive factor (ISF), can profoundly suppress the full range of immune responses. Normal adult cells do not produce this powerful protein—but incredibly, researchers have found that it *is* produced by fetal cells.

Like the fetus, tumor cells can also stimulate the body to produce suppressor T cells, which then shut off any response directed against the tumor. Laboratory mice with tumors have been shown to have an abnormally high number of suppressor T cells in their spleens; when researchers remove the spleens, these animals exhibit much longer survival times. Treatments that interrupt normal suppressor T cell functions have also extended the survival time of mice with certain kinds of tumors. These findings suggest that in the absence of suppressor T cells, the immune system can exert its full force against the cancer cells. Although the mechanisms at work are not well understood, both tumor cells and the fetus may stimulate the production of host suppressor T cells by manipulating lymphokine signals. And there is the possibility that, by understanding the nature of these suppressor lymphokines, we may yet uncover ways to restore normal suppressor T cell levels in cancer patients, thereby enabling the immune system to turn the full power of its attack against tumor cells.

Many researchers believe that knowledge gained from the study of the relationship between mother and fetus will aid in the search for more precise and effective treatments against cancer. The insights provided by reproductive immunology will then have given us new power not only to help create life by curing infertility and the diseases of pregnancy, but also to preserve life.

nine

THE BATTLE AGAINST SELF

I knew that I myself was very strange to me. I thrust forth a hand to regard it. I did not, in the deepest sense, know whose hand it was.

ROBERT PENN WARREN,
A Place to Come to

Perhaps the greatest wonder of the human immune system is the breadth of its arsenal. Helper and killer T cells can recognize and respond to an estimated one million different antigens. B cells are programmed to produce antibodies against the same astonishing number of foreign cells and substances—including antibodies that can target all sorts of odd, artificially created substances never encountered by the body before. Over the course of its evolution, the immune system has come to recognize and react swiftly and surely against a staggering number of potentially dangerous cells and substances. Diversity of response is absolutely critical to survival. But there is an equally critical limitation on the activities of the immune system. For while it must be able to react against the vast range of foreign antigens, the immune system must *not* react against self antigens—those molecules that are carried on the cells of the body itself. Any substance, natural or synthetic, self or non-self, is capable of triggering an immune response once it is recognized by the immune system. Immunologists speak of a state of *immune tolerance,* the condition in which the cells of the immune system do not react destructively against the antigens on cells that make up the tissues and organs of the body.

Immune tolerance develops early in an infant's life. Although the exact process by which immune cells learn to distinguish self from non-self is not clearly understood, the importance of immune tolerance—standing as the only barrier between the body and the destructive force of the immune system—is quite clear. When immune tolerance breaks down, in certain rare cases, the immune system turns on the body itself, ferociously attacking and destroying cells of the kidneys, heart, brain, or other organs and tissues.

This aberrant form of immune response, called *autoimmunity,* is literally a form of immunologic self-destruction. Once an autoimmune response is initiated, it is carried forward with the same intensity and force as an immune response against any foreign pathogen. Killer T cells and antibodies target the body's own cells. Phagocytes engulf and destroy bits and pieces of host tissue. And unless the attack is stopped with immunosuppressive drugs or radiation therapy, these tissues will be relentlessly destroyed.

A wide variety of diseases are autoimmune in nature. Multiple sclerosis, rheumatoid arthritis, systemic lupus erythematosus, myasthenia gravis, Hashimoto's disease, and a number of other diseases all represent autoimmune disorders. In fact, no tissue or organ of the body is spared the possibility of a self-destructive attack. In multiple sclerosis, the immune system turns against the tissues of the central nervous system. In rheumatoid arthritis, the tissues of the joints come under attack. In myasthenia gravis, it is the voluntary muscles; in Hashimoto's disease, the thyroid gland; in systemic lupus erythematosus, the brain, kidneys, lungs, skin, and joints may all be attacked and severely damaged. Underlying each of these diseases is a fundamental breakdown in the ability of the immune system to distinguish between self and non-self, friend and foe.

At the turn of the century, the great microbiologist Paul Ehrlich proposed the first theory of autoimmunity, or "horror autotoxicus," as he described it. In a healthy state, the immune system does not destroy the cells that make up the body. It follows, Ehrlich reasoned, that in normal circumstances the cells of the immune system simply do not react to self antigens. Only in extremely rare cases would immune cells emerge that recognize and react against the body itself, and the result was autoimmune disease.

For many years, Ehrlich's theory of autoimmunity held sway. Autoreactive immune cells, cells which reacted against host tissue, came to be called *forbidden clones*. Most immunologists believed that when these autoreactive cells happened to appear, an ever-alert immune surveillance system swiftly detected and destroyed them. Only when the system broke down, and autoreactive cells were allowed to survive, would autoimmune responses occur.

In the last decade, immunologists have discovered that Ehrlich's hypothesis of autoimmunity is only partially correct. The results of recent studies indicate that certain potentially harmful autoreactive cells are indeed selectively destroyed by the immune system, especially during an individual's early life. But Ehrlich was mistaken in his assumption that the emergence and survival of autoreactive cells is a rare event that always dooms the body to immunologic self-destruction.

One of the revolutionary discoveries of modern immunology, in fact, is that the nature of self and non-self recognition is far more complex than had been previously thought. The appearance of immune cells that react to self antigens is not a rare occurrence, as Ehrlich believed; in fact, T and B cells which recognize self antigens are *always* present in the adult immune system. And some of these cells, in particular killer T cells, actually use their powers of self-recognition in the battle against infectious viruses. In order for a killer T cell to destroy a virally infected cell, it must recognize not only the viral antigens that appear on the cell's surface, but also specific self antigens that identify the invaded cell as self. In effect, the T cell must be able to recognize self and non-self simultaneously. Otherwise, it is unable to target the invaded cell for attack. Although a killer T cell may be targeted specifically against host cells infected with influenza virus, for example, it will not kill cells of another individual infected with the identical viral strain. The ability of T cells to recognize self, rather than constituting a defect of immune response, appears to be absolutely essential in the normal functioning of the immune system.

With these findings, the fundamental questions surrounding autoimmunity have changed. Ehrlich wondered what might allow for the rare appearance of autoreactive cells. Today immunologists recognize that these cells are always present, and the important question now concerns how they are prevented from expressing their destructive autoimmune potential. The key to understanding the control of self and non-self recognition appears to lie in the mechanisms that normally suppress the activities of latent but potentially dangerous autoreactive cells.

Research into the disorders that represent a breakdown of these mechanisms—the wide spectrum of autoimmune syndromes—may provide some clues. It now seems clear, for example, that the causes of autoimmune disease are as complex as the nature of autoimmunity itself. Most diseases have a single primary cause—a virus, bacterium, or some other pathogen. But gathering evidence suggests that autoimmune diseases are the result not of a single factor but the relatively rare convergence of several factors.

One of the earliest insights into the nature of autoimmunity came as a curious sidelight to Pasteur's work on a rabies vaccine. In 1885, Pasteur developed the vaccine by injecting attenuated rabies viruses into spinal cord tissue from laboratory rabbits, and then inoculating patients with the infected tissue. Pasteur's vaccine saved lives; but soon after the technique entered clinical practice, reports began to appear of patients who had developed acute paralysis shortly after immunization with the vaccine. Investigators were shocked by the severity of the unexplained reactions. Some researchers suggested that the paralysis was caused by the attenuated viruses themselves. Others believed that the injected spinal cord tissue was somehow responsible. For more than forty years, the exact cause of the rare phenomenon remained unknown.

Then, in the 1930s, a group of American researchers performed a simple experiment that provided the answer. They injected laboratory monkeys with tissue from the nervous systems of rabbits—tissue from which all viruses had been removed. A short time later, several of the monkeys developed symptoms of nervous system damage almost identical to those seen after injections of the rabies virus vaccine. The experiment proved that the tissue itself, and not a virus, was responsible for the rare central nervous system destruction that followed rabies vaccination. And the researchers guessed correctly that the injected tissue, because of its foreign antigens, was triggering an immune response—but a response that was not limited to the rabbit tissue. The foreign tissue antigens had elicited an immune response that also turned against the central nervous system of the monkeys themselves. This discovery led researchers to an even more important observation: the disease that had been induced experimentally, which came to be called *experimental encephalomyelitis,* was almost identical in its symptoms to a naturally occurring disease—multiple sclerosis.

Multiple sclerosis is also a disease of the central nervous system. Its symptoms include numbness, hand tremors, loss of coordination and balance, difficulty in speaking, and, in severe cases, paralysis. These symptoms, which usually occur intermittently but with increasing severity, are the result of the autoimmune destruction of an important component of nerve tissue. In the central nervous system, nerve cells possess long extensions called *axons* that make contact with other nerve cells. Axons are wrapped in several protective layers of a material called *myelin.* Both experimental encephalomyelitis and multiple sclerosis involve an acute or chronic inflammatory response that leads to the breakdown of this myelin sheath, a process called *demyelination.* The destruction of the myelin sheath causes the formation of scar tissue, which then disrupts nerve transmissions, resulting in the similar symptoms of the two diseases.

With the discovery of experimental encephalomyelitis, researchers had found a useful animal model for multiple sclerosis. And in the years that followed, the study of experimental encephalomyelitis would yield several important insights into the nature of the disease it so closely resembled. In the 1960s, researchers found that the experimental disease was mediated by T cells, confirming its immunologic nature. When they isolated T cells from animals that had been immunized with nerve tissue and then injected the cells into untreated animals, these naive animals began to develop the symptoms of experimental encephalomyelitis. During the same period, investigators identified a single protein in myelin, called *myelin basic protein,* which by itself is capable of triggering the same autoimmune response as the crude preparations of nerve tissue. With this discovery, researchers had isolated a fundamental component of the disease process. Myelin basic protein is one of the major antigens of nerve tissue against which the immune system reacts in experimental encephalomyelitis. When investigators added myelin basic protein to cultures of sensitized T cells taken from laboratory animals, they found that the T cells were stimulated to grow and to release migration inhibitory factor. The events are characteristic of inflammatory responses, and their presence proves that myelin basic protein is indeed a key trigger of experimental encephalomyelitis.

Investigators compared these findings with results obtained with the immune cells of multiple sclerosis patients. They isolated T cells from patients with the disease and incubated them with myelin basic protein. The T cells began to proliferate and release migration inhibitory factor—the same T cell responses that took place in the experimental disease. It was now clear that the immunologic processes of the two diseases were very similar. In both, myelin tissue is damaged or destroyed. This tissue damage is mediated by T cells and macrophages. And in both diseases, myelin basic protein appears to be the major antigenic trigger.

But there are important differences as well. In multiple sclerosis, the breakdown of myelin is chronic, persisting for years. In experimental encephalomyelitis, however, the inflammation is acute, reaching a peak and then subsiding. Animals that survive the acute inflammation rarely have any subsequent symptoms of the disease. Researchers knew how to cause the experimental disease, of course; but they had no idea what caused naturally occurring multiple sclerosis. Why did the immune system in multiple sclerosis suddenly react against myelin basic protein? What sustained the autoimmune response once it began?

Most researchers believed that the prolonged nature of the disease process held the key to uncovering the cause of multiple sclerosis. The experimental model had taught them a great deal about the disease process, but now they would have to search elsewhere for an answer. And one trail led them to a virus.

In 1953, investigating the geographic distribution of multiple sclerosis, Dr. Leonard Kurland discovered an intriguing fact. The disease, he observed, was significantly more prevalent in temperate climates than in tropical or subtropical regions. The incidence of multiple sclerosis was three times higher in Nova

Scotia, for example, than in New Orleans, and thirty-seven times higher in Minneapolis than in Mexico City. Indeed, the farther one moved from the equator, the greater the apparent risk of contracting multiple sclerosis. Later investigations turned up other provocative facts. When children under the age of fifteen moved from a low risk area to a high risk area, they took on the risk factor of their new environment. A young child moving from New Orleans to Nova Scotia would have an increased risk of contracting multiple sclerosis. A child moving from Minneapolis to Mexico City would have a decreased risk of contracting the disease. But when individuals over the age of fifteen moved from one geographic risk area to another, their chances of contracting the disease did not change.

Epidemiologists compared Kurland's findings on multiple sclerosis with those of other known diseases, and they discovered an interesting link. The incidence of measles infections was related, in a curious way, to the geographic distribution of multiple sclerosis. Measles infections tend to occur early in life in tropical and subtropical areas, and later in life in temperate climates. And a majority of multiple sclerosis patients had contracted measles infections later in life than did the general population. Could there be some connection between contracting measles at an older age and the development of multiple sclerosis? Was there in fact a link with the measles virus?

Certainly the precedent for such a link existed. In 1926, researchers reported seven cases of acute encephalitis (inflammation of the brain) in patients who had received routine smallpox vaccinations. Within the next few years, investigators reported more cases of acute encephalitis following not only smallpox but also measles and chickenpox infections. It was clear that viruses could induce inflammation of the brain.

Could a chronic measles virus infection be responsible for the prolonged autoimmune inflammatory responses of multiple sclerosis?

In 1962, researchers discovered that antimeasles antibody levels in the blood and spinal fluid of multiple sclerosis patients were higher than normal—another piece of evidence that suggested a link between the measles virus and multiple sclerosis. Even more significant, investigators at Long Island College Hospital found the presence of measles virus antigens in the gastrointestinal tract of each of thirty-six multiple sclerosis patients they examined. While these findings are provocative, however, they are by no means final proof that the measles virus is a cause of multiple sclerosis. One important piece of evidence is still missing. For despite intensive efforts, investigators have not yet been able to demonstrate the presence of the measles virus in patients with multiple sclerosis.

Some researchers claim that the failure to find the measles virus casts doubt over the hypothesis that the virus is indeed linked to multiple sclerosis. But there could well be other reasons for this failure. The measles virus may be present in these patients in a latent or defective form, perhaps in a state in which it is no longer able to replicate. The herpes virus, for example, which has been studied extensively in its active form, has never been observed in its latent form. Scientists have almost no idea what the latent herpes virus looks like or how it functions during its latent stage. The measles virus may also exist in multiple sclerosis patients in a form we cannot yet identify. Researchers simply do not know.

Still, the hypothesis of a viral connection to multiple sclerosis is a strong one; and it has been strengthened by the discovery of another important link between a virus and an autoimmune disorder—rheumatoid arthritis.

In rheumatoid arthritis, cells of the immune system swarm into the tissues of the joints, attacking and destroying connective tissue and even bone. Virtually every immunologic weapon is activated against the body. Phagocytes, killer T cells, antibodies, and complement proteins are all involved in the destruction of joint tissue. Nonimmune cells in the joints release a variety of potent substances that add to the destructive process. The autoimmune attack in rheumatoid arthritis even turns against antibodies themselves. Patients with the disease produce circulating autoantibodies, called *rheumatoid factors,* which target other antibodies. These autoantibodies bind with circulating antibodies, forming antibody-autoantibody complexes that are a major contributing factor in the disease process.

Immunologists know a great deal about the details of this highly complex disease, including the role that lymphokines play in initiating and amplifying the damaging inflammation of rheumatoid arthritis. But while we understand the mechanisms at work, we do not understand fully what sets these mechanisms off in the first place—what initiates the violent autoimmune response.

In 1976, researchers Margaret Alspaugh and Eng Tan discovered a curious relationship between rheumatoid arthritis and the Epstein-Barr virus, which may someday provide an answer. Epstein-Barr virus is known to cause infectious mononucleosis. And there is growing evidence that this virus may also be related to two forms of cancer: Burkitt's lymphoma and nasopharnygeal carcinoma. Alspaugh and Tan found that an unusually high number of rheumatoid arthritis patients had antibodies in their blood specifically targeted to an antigen normally found only on cells infected by the Epstein-Barr virus.

The discovery was startling. The vast majority of blood samples from healthy individuals do not contain this antibody. Clearly, a significant number of rheumatoid arthritis patients have been exposed to Epstein-Barr virus infections.

Epstein-Barr virus targets B cells. When human B cells are placed in a sterile laboratory dish and incubated with this virus, the B cells undergo a dramatic change. Instead of dying within a few days, as normal B cells would, the infected cells are transformed into cells that can live and reproduce indefinitely. Like spontaneously arising cancer cells, B cells infected by the Epstein-Barr virus are "immortalized." They will grow and divide as long as they are supplied with proper nutrients. Some researchers suspect that its ability to immortalize B cells may be how the Epstein-Barr virus causes cancer.

When researchers studied B cells infected by Epstein-Barr virus, they also discovered that these immortalized cells continue to produce and release antibodies. Each infected B cell produces the specific antibody it has been genetically programmed to synthesize. And some of these antibodies are autoantibodies—the very same autoantibodies that are produced by patients with rheumatoid arthritis.

This discovery forged an important link between Epstein-Barr virus and rheumatoid arthritis. But it also raised a puzzling question. Many people are exposed to Epstein-Barr virus, just as they are to the measles virus, but only a relatively few develop serious autoimmune disorders like rheumatoid arthritis or multiple sclerosis. Most Epstein-Barr virus infections are successfully controlled by the immune system. If Epstein-Barr virus is indeed the culprit in rheumatoid arthritis, there has to be some reason why it causes such destruction only in certain individuals. Researchers began to wonder if a defect in the immune responses of rheumatoid arthritis patients prevents them from defending themselves against a chronic infection by the virus.

To test this possibility, researchers isolated T and B cells from healthy individuals and from rheumatoid arthritis patients. The cells were then infected with Epstein-Barr virus. When investigators compared the responses of these two groups of cells, they found a dramatic difference. In the cultures of healthy cells, B cells produced increasing amounts of antibodies for about ten days, and then antibody production dramatically dropped off. But the production of antibodies by the B cells of rheumatoid arthritis patients did not slow; the virally infected cells continued to produce increasing quantities of antibodies for several days after the cells from normal individuals had stopped. Obviously some mechanism for the suppression of antibody production, operating in mixtures of healthy T and B cells, was absent in the cells of rheumatoid arthritis patients.

In order to narrow their investigation, researchers removed T cells from the cultures to see if they might be responsible for the suppression. Isolated B cells from healthy individuals were infected with Epstein-Barr virus. And without the presence of T cells, the healthy B cells showed no decrease in antibody production after ten days—exactly the response that had been seen in B cells from rheumatoid arthritis patients. When healthy T cells were added to the broth, however, antibody production began to slow. Clearly, healthy T cells exert some kind of control over the B-cell production of antibody. To confirm this finding, researchers added T cells from patients with rheumatoid arthritis to the B cell cultures. The level of antibody production continued unabated; the normal control mechanism was absent.

These findings were conclusive. While healthy T cells are able to suppress abnormal antibody production induced by Epstein-Barr virus infection, T cells from rheumatoid arthritis patients lack this ability. Some researchers believe the Epstein-Barr virus, by infecting B cells, may actually trigger the onset of rheumatoid arthritis. Others believe that the virus may simply be a factor in perpetuating the autoimmune responses associated with the disease. But perhaps the most interesting discovery to emerge from the research is that the Epstein-Barr virus, if it is indeed a factor in the disease, does not work alone. A congenital defect in the function of T cells appears to serve as the predisposing factor that allows the Epstein-Barr virus, when it invades, to generate autoimmune responses.

A dysfunction of lymphocytes also appears to be a factor in the development of another serious autoimmune disorder, *systemic lupus erythematosus,* or SLE. In patients with the disease, B cells appear to be totally out of control. They proliferate at a heightened rate and manufacture high levels of virtually all types of antibodies. Large numbers of circulating autoantibodies are produced which can recognize a variety of host antigens. Deposited along blood vessels and in the kidneys, these autoantibodies attract macrophages, T cells, and other cells capable of causing widespread tissue damage. B cells in SLE patients have even been shown to produce autoantibodies that target host T and B cells. The result, in extreme cases of the disease, can be serious kidney, liver, and central nervous system destruction.

Immunologists do not understand why the normal controls

on the functioning of B cells have broken down in these patients. The delicate balance between the ability of B cells to produce antibodies and the ability of suppressor T cells to control the activity of B cells may have broken down in patients with SLE. But one intriguing aspect of the disease has led scientists to some important discoveries. Systemic lupus erythematosus, like rheumatoid arthritis, myasthenia gravis, and many other autoimmune disorders, strikes women far more often than it does men. Approximately 90 percent of all patients with SLE are women—and during the childbearing years, the ratio of women to men with the disease can be as high as twenty to one.

In the 1950s, researchers discovered an animal model for SLE that would help them investigate the reasons why women are at greater risk of developing the disease. A special inbred strain of mice called New Zealand B/W mice was found to be particularly susceptible to a disease whose symptoms and incidence were strikingly similar to those of systemic lupus erythematosus. Like human patients with SLE, many of these mice developed destructive inflammation of the kidneys. Examination of the diseased organs revealed the presence of the same kind of antibody-autoantibody complexes that are seen in human SLE. Moreover, female mice were found to be far more susceptible to the disease than males.

To test the possibility that male and female hormones might play some role in the development of the SLE-like disease, researchers devised a series of experiments to measure the effects of these hormones in B/W mice. They began by neutering a group of mice prior to puberty, in order to interrupt normal hormone production. The male mice were then given estrogens, female sex hormones, and the female mice were given androgens, male sex hormones. During the next few months, the treated male mice began to develop the SLE-like disease in greater numbers and with more severe symptoms than had been seen in normal male mice. And female mice given male hormones had a dramatically *lower* incidence and severity of the disease than their normal female counterparts.

These experiments provided compelling evidence that male and female hormones were able to alter significantly the course of the autoimmune disease in mice. And clinical observations suggest that hormones may play an equally important role in the development of human SLE. In 1978, for example, researchers noted that the use of oral contraceptives, composed of female sex hormones, aggravate symptoms of the disease in patients with SLE. Women in their childbearing years, a time when the level of female sex hormones is at its peak, demonstrate the highest overall incidence of the disease. And men with abnormally high levels of the female hormone estradiol have been found to have a higher incidence of SLE than normal males.

How sex hormones contribute to the development and progress of the disease has yet to be determined, although researchers have recently made some fascinating observations. Alfred Steinberg and his colleagues at the National Institutes of Health have discovered that male hormones appear to favor the development of suppressor T cells in the thymus, while female hormones tend to favor the development of helper T cells. The increased production of suppressor T cells in males may be a key factor in controlling growth and antibody production of the hyperactive B cells characteristic of SLE patients.

The balance of male and female hormones appears to be a significant factor in rheumatoid arthritis, myasthenia gravis,

Hashimoto's disease, and a number of other disorders. But sex hormones do not appear to be a factor in all autoimmune diseases. In multiple sclerosis, for example, the risk of contracting the disease is equal for males and females.

This evidence suggests that while all autoimmune diseases result from the convergence of a number of factors, the specific nature and role of these factors vary among the different forms of autoimmune responses. And yet there does appear to be a single factor which may play a role in all autoimmune disorders, as well as many other forms of disease: a predisposition for developing certain diseases that is programmed into our genes from birth.

In 1964, F. Lilly and his colleagues were engaged in experiments on the susceptibility of certain mice to a leukemia-causing virus called the Gross virus. Drawn from several different inbred strains, the mice differed widely in their pattern of histocompatibility antigens (the antigens that control graft acceptance or rejection). Lilly began to notice that only certain strains of mice—those that shared a common set of histocompatibility antigens—when injected with the Gross virus, went on to develop leukemia. Mice of an inbred strain with histocompatibility type k were extremely susceptible to Gross virus infection, for example, while mice of an unrelated histocompatibility type b were virtually resistant.

These observations were startling in their implications. The ultimate fate of the infected laboratory mice, survival or destruction, appeared to depend on the presence or absence of specific forms of a small group of cell surface antigens whose synthesis was dictated by a select group of genes previously linked to the control of graft rejection. In the intensive search that followed the release of Lilly's findings, researchers discovered that a significant number of virally induced cancers were related to the presence of certain histocompatibility genes in laboratory animals.

And before long, a connection was found between specific histocompatibility genes and a human disease—*ankylosing spondylitis,* a chronic inflammatory disease that occurs at the sites where ligaments attach to bone. Genetic predisposition to the disease had long been recognized; more than half of all patients with ankylosing spondylitis have family members who are also afflicted. In 1973, two research groups discovered how susceptibility to the disease might be inherited. They found that the statistical probability of developing ankylosing spondylitis is markedly higher in people who have a particular form of one histocompatibility gene, designated HLA-B27. Over 90 percent of all patients with the disease have this particular gene, contrasted with about 7 percent of the general population.

In the years that followed, researchers uncovered links between a number of other diseases and the presence of certain forms of specific histocompatibility genes. Individuals with the histocompatibility genes HLA-Dw4 and HLA-DR4, for example, are at much greater risk of developing rheumatoid arthritis. Multiple sclerosis, myasthenia gravis, Hashimoto's disease, and systemic lupus erythematosus have all been related to specific sets of histocompatibility genes.

Histocompatibility genes were first discovered during research into graft rejection. These genes contain the information for producing specific proteins which can act as extremely potent antigenic triggers of graft rejection. But this property is only an incidental function of histocompatibility antigens, in the very rare case of a tissue or organ transplant. In the normal workings of an immune cell, histocompatibility antigens serve a number of other important purposes. Some of the genes, for example, contain the information for producing antigens that determine how cells of the immune system will respond to particular foreign antigens.

Immunologists and geneticists have developed a large variety of inbred strains of laboratory mice distinguished by their unique pattern of immune responses to specific antigens. One strain of inbred mice will respond very actively to an antigen found in chick eggs; a different strain will not respond at all. By careful genetic analysis of these mice, researchers have discovered a specific group of histocompatibility genes, called *immune response genes.* These genes contain the instructions for producing proteins that allow T and B cells to recognize and respond in a certain way to a specific foreign antigen. One form of an immune response gene will permit the activation of helper T cells and antibody production that are essential for a vigorous immune response against a specific antigen. An alternate form of the same immune response gene will promote the production of suppressor T cells that can block the generation of a strong immune response.

Some researchers believe that particular forms of these histocompatibility genes may, in the same way, predispose certain individuals to autoimmune responses by inadvertently permitting the immune system to mistake host antigens as foreign. A number of host antigens happen to resemble very closely certain antigens that appear on bacteria, viruses, and other infectious organisms. In most cases, immune response genes permit T cells to recognize only the antigens that are *unique* to a pathogen. But in other cases, a different form of immune response gene may permit T cells to recognize these look-alike, or *cross-reactive,* antigens found on both the pathogen and host cells. In reacting against the pathogen, T cells will also react against the look-alike antigens on the body's own cells, initiating an autoimmune response. In the case of multiple sclerosis, for example, it is quite possible that a certain form of immune response gene permits T cells and antibodies to recognize not only the pathogen that initiated their activation, but also the myelin sheath surrounding nerve cells—because an antigen on this sheath looks like an antigen on the pathogen.

This phenomenon of *molecular mimicry* is known to play an important role in rheumatic fever. The disease is initiated by group A streptococci, the same strain of bacteria that causes strep throat and scarlet fever. In most cases, these infections are successfully resolved by the immune system. But in a relatively small percentage of individuals, untreated strep infections can lead to rheumatic fever—a serious disease in which the immune system turns against tissues of the joints, heart, skin, kidneys, brain, and other organs. These tissues happen to bear antigens that mimic specific antigens on group A streptococci. In general, immune response genes do not permit immune cells to recognize these cross-reactive antigens. When a certain form of an immune response gene happens to permit this recognition, however, a defensive response against the invading pathogen becomes an attack against self, and rheumatic fever results.

There is also evidence that normally distinct self antigens may be modified to look like foreign antigens during the course of an infection. Kidney and heart tissues bear antigens that resemble those of group A streptococci, but they are usually found in a buried or cryptic form not easily recognized by the immune system. A strep infection may result in the release of certain inflammatory substances, however, which chemically modify these antigens. And in individuals whose immune-response genes permit the recognition of the modified antigens, an autoimmune response may be generated.

Viruses like the measles or Epstein-Barr virus may indirectly cause the conversion of self into non-self in much the same manner. The process of a viral infection, or even the immune response against virally infected cells, may in some way modify specific host antigens, especially those found on cell membranes. And the slightest change in shape, or the removal of a small fragment from a cell surface antigen, can quickly transform it from self into non-self. In certain individuals, a precise form of the immune response gene will permit T and B cells to recognize these altered antigens as foreign, triggering an autoimmune attack. Many researchers believe that the presence of chronic viral infections may maintain the level of such altered antigens, resulting in the prolonged nature of autoimmune diseases like multiple sclerosis and rheumatoid arthritis.

Current research seems to indicate that a number of autoimmune disorders may be initiated by infectious agents like viruses and bacteria. But these pathogens can only trigger autoimmune responses in those individuals already predisposed by other factors. In rheumatoid arthritis, for example, a defect in the mechanism by which T cells control B cell production of antibodies may serve as the primary predisposing factor. This defect will pose no problem until the Epstein-Barr virus invades B cells, and the genetic defect is expressed. Sex hormones may then play a role in determining the progress of the disease, perhaps by changing the balance of suppressor and helper T cells and their regulation of B cell growth and antibody production. Underlying all of these factors is a predisposition to autoimmune disease that appears to be programmed into an individual's immune response genes. Alone, any one of these factors would most likely not trigger an autoimmune disease; only with the rare convergence of a number of factors do autoimmune responses occur.

There is still much to be learned about the fundamental nature of self and non-self recognition and its dysfunction in autoimmune disorders. Autoimmunity remains one of the great unsolved mysteries—the "black box" of immunology, as some investigators have called it. Still, the insights we have gained into the process and probable cause of various autoimmune disorders are important in their own right. Even isolated breakthroughs in understanding may soon lead to dramatic new ways to treat and perhaps even prevent these devastating disorders.

The evidence that infectious agents like the measles virus and Epstein-Barr virus can trigger autoimmune responses, for example, suggests that vaccines against these viruses may be of use in preventing certain forms of autoimmunity. Indeed, just such a vaccine may already be at work. In 1966, the United States initiated the measles immunization program, and researchers have been following the subsequent incidence of multiple sclerosis with great interest. If the measles virus indeed plays some role in initiating this disease, then epidemiologists should begin to notice a decline in the number of new cases of multiple sclerosis in the coming years. These findings would, of course, encourage the development of vaccines against other pathogens suspected of inducing autoimmune responses. And new information about the role of genetic factors in autoimmunity may help physicians identify individuals at greatest risk of developing certain disorders, so that preventive vaccines could be effectively targeted.

For patients with autoimmune disease, the most promising treatment lies in the potential use of lymphokines. Research into the role lymphokines play in rheumatoid arthritis, for example, suggests that immunologists may be able to modify the course of the disease by controlling the activity of a single lymphokine: interleukin 1.

Rheumatoid arthritis is marked by an explosion of immunologic activity directed against the tissues of the joints. Macrophages, T cells, and antibodies flood into these tissues, targeting host cells for destruction. T cells release a lymphokine called *osteoclast activating factor,* which in normal circumstances is involved in the routine maintenance of bone structure; but in the autoimmune responses of rheumatoid arthritis, abnormally high concentrations of this lymphokine begin to cause the actual destruction of bone. Chemotactic factors, released by both macrophages and T cells, recruit growing numbers of immune cells to participate in the destruction; macrophages even enlist certain nonimmune cells that are found within the joints themselves to join in an autoimmune attack which appears to be virtually out of control.

But the cells involved in the autoimmune responses of rheumatoid arthritis are not out of control. In fact, they appear to be largely under the controlling influence of a single immune cell, using a single lymphokine signal.

Since the 1940s, researchers have known that patients with rheumatoid arthritis produce autoantibodies that target antibodies normally circulating in the blood. The binding of these autoantibodies with normal antibodies produces immune complexes, which appear to stimulate macrophages to release interleukin 1, as well as their full arsenal of inflammatory substances. Interleukin 1 then triggers the release of interleukin 2, and sets off the lymphokine cycle that activates and amplifies the autoimmune responses of T cells, B cells, and macrophages.

But the production of interleukin 1 plays another role as well. In 1976, Jean-Michel Dayer and Stephen Krane at Massachusetts General Hospital in Boston isolated a group of specialized cells found in relatively small numbers in the tissues of the joints. These cells, called *synovial cells,* perform a number of functions in healthy tissue. But when Dayer and Krane isolated synovial cells from rheumatoid arthritis patients, they found that these cells, unlike the cells from healthy individuals, produced extremely high levels of inflammatory substances like prostaglandins and collagenase, an enzyme that breaks down connective tissue. These substances were known to play a dominant role in the destruction of tissue and the pain associated with rheumatoid arthritis. But curiously, when synovial cells were left in laboratory dishes over a prolonged period of time, the cells gradually lost their ability to produce inflammatory substances. Dayer and Krane supposed that some factor present in the environment of the joint must stimulate the release of these substances—a factor that was absent when the cells were left in laboratory dishes. They wondered if the stimulating factor might be a lymphokine.

The researchers removed broth from a culture of lymphocytes and macrophages and added it to a culture of synovial cells that had stopped producing inflammatory substances. Within a few days, the synovial cells were once again releasing high levels of prostaglandins and collagenase. Dayer and Krane had confirmed that a factor in the broth was responsible for stimulating these cells to participate in the inflammatory response. Later, in a collaborative effort with investigators at the National Institutes of Health in Maryland, Dayer and Krane made the startling discovery that the stimulating factor was, in fact, interleukin 1. At the time, interleukin 1 was thought to act only on immune cells. But now there was compelling evidence that it has a powerful effect on nonimmune synovial cells as well.

Indeed, by releasing interleukin 1, the macrophage apparently serves as the controlling force behind almost all of the inflammatory responses associated with rheumatoid arthritis. Virtually the entire range of cells involved in the autoimmune attack—T cells, B cells, and synovial cells—are under the control of the macrophage.

These findings may soon lead to a revolutionary treatment for rheumatoid arthritis. If interleukin 1 is indeed the critical link in the self-destructive chain reaction, then drugs that block its action, called interleukin 1 *antagonists,* should be able to stop the autoimmune response at its source. Without the presence of interleukin 1, T cells, B cells, and synovial cells would lack an important signal they need to begin the inflammatory process. Research is currently underway to develop effective interleukin 1 antagonists.

Other lymphokines may prove to be of value in treating other autoimmune disorders. Many researchers believe that suppressor T cells work by releasing certain as yet unidentified suppressor lymphokines. In the near future, immunologists may learn how to administer these lymphokines therapeutically in order to slow down or stop autoimmune responses. In SLE, for example, a defect either in the number of suppressor T cells or in their ability to produce suppressor lymphokines appears to allow B cells to proliferate and produce antibodies beyond the normal control of the immune system. By administering lymphokines that signal B cells to slow down their activity, immunologists may eventually be able to control the autoimmune responses of SLE—and thereby offer the first specific and effective treatment for the disease.

As scientists learn more about the mechanisms that control normal immune responses, we will come to understand better the fundamental factors that influence the breakdown of immunologic functions in autoimmune disorders. And armed with this understanding, immunologists may uncover new and powerful ways to control the behavior of the immune system when it moves from defense to self-destruction.

ten

THE IgE CONNECTION

At this point an unforeseen event occurred.

CHARLES RICHET, 1913

Thirty-five million Americans suffer from allergies—everything from the runny nose and watery eyes of hay fever to severe complications brought on by insect bites or adverse reactions to certain drugs. Allergies can be deadly serious: acute asthmatic attacks are the cause of as many as six thousand deaths every year; anaphylactic shock, the most severe of all allergic reactions, claims several hundred victims annually. And yet in each allergic reaction, the body's enemy is not an invading microorganism at all, but a perfectly commonplace substance. Pollen, dust, animal dander, and even certain foods—substances which, in and of themselves, are completely harmless —can all trigger allergic reactions. When the immune system responds against them as it would against a microbial enemy, however, immune responses themselves can cause serious symptoms and suffering.

Medical researchers have long known that allergic reactions are associated with the body's immune system, but the exact nature of that association and the precise physiologic details of an allergic reaction have revealed themselves only in the last twenty years. And the unraveling of the mystery has involved the piecing together of clues gathered by a number of investigators over many years.

The English physician Charles Harrison Blackley, working during the last half of the nineteenth century, conducted the first truly scientific studies of allergy. Blackley suffered from hay fever; and like many researchers of his time, he conducted his experiments on himself—perhaps in part because his patients with hay fever, as anxious as they were for a cure, may not have been quite as willing as Blackley to suffer in its pursuit.

Blackley knew of the several hypotheses in vogue at the time, each of which attempted to explain the cause of hay fever. The hypotheses implicated everything from the influence of light and heat to dust, the action of ozone, certain odors, and the inhalation of pollen grains. Blackley began his experiments by exposing himself to each of these substances individually, in order to test their possible role in hay fever. The real culprit, he soon discovered, was pollen. (Later, moving a vase of dried grasses from one room to another in his house and inadvertently releasing their pollens, Blackley confirmed his observations.)

Collecting pollens from over eighty different plants, Blackley inhaled them, applied them to the inner surface of his eyelids, and scratched them into his skin to see how powerful each was in producing the symptoms of hay fever. Inhaled grass pollens seemed to produce the strongest effect, sometimes even causing a serious asthmatic attack. And Blackley observed that when he scratched his skin with any of the pollens that activated his hay fever, the area quickly became reddened and swollen. Pollens that did not activate his hay fever, he found, also did not produce the distinctive skin reaction.

Blackley invented several ingenious methods to measure the number of pollen grains in the air. He even devised a way to measure pollen counts as high as two thousand feet above the ground by using sticky glass slides attached to kites. The daily pollen counts correlated closely with the severity of his own hay fever symptoms. As little as 0.00000007 ounce of pollen inhaled during a 24-hour period was enough to induce hay fever. The ability of pollen grains themselves to cause hay fever was not related to their individual size, Blackley discovered, but to the relative content of certain substances, later called *allergens*, released by the pollen.

Blackley's observations laid the foundation for modern research into the nature of allergy and asthma. His investigations were followed, in the first years of the twentieth century, by the work of two French researchers, Charles Richet and Paul Portier. Visiting an area of the French Mediterranean where large populations of sea anemone and Portuguese man-of-war posed a threat to swimmers, the researchers wondered if it might be possible to immunize against the potent toxins secreted by these creatures. To test their idea, they injected laboratory dogs with small doses of sea anemone toxin, and after a time injected a second small dose. The results could not have been more unexpected. Several of the dogs were quickly thrown into convulsions and respiratory collapse. Within hours they were dead. Richet and Portier repeated the experiment, with the same puzzling and disturbing outcome: a number of the dogs, injected with the second dose of toxin, promptly went into shock and died.

The researchers had no explanation for what had occurred. The amounts of toxin they had administered were too small to be lethal in themselves. According to everything that was known, the injections should have resulted in a form of protective immunity against the sea anemone toxin.

Richet and Portier named the puzzling reaction *anaphylaxis* (without or against protection). The term distinguished this fatal response from the expected *prophylactic* or protective effect of immunization. Anaphylaxis was clearly immunologic in nature. *Any* foreign substance, administered in a certain way, could produce the lethal reaction when the first and second injections were separated by at least seven to ten days. And like other immune responses, the anaphylactic response was specific. It occurred only in animals that had been previously sensitized to the injected substance. The period between the first and second injections apparently gave the body an opportunity to develop some unknown form of immunity against the antigen. Without this previous sensitivity, the anaphylactic response would not occur.

In many ways, the anaphylactic response appeared to obey the same basic immunologic rules as another immune response —the Koch phenomenon of delayed-type hypersensitivity. But in one crucial way these two responses were quite different. Using tuberculin antigen, Robert Koch had demonstrated that an inflammatory skin reaction required at least 24 to 48 hours to reach its peak. The anaphylactic reaction occurred much more swiftly, sometimes within minutes after the second injection. For that reason, anaphylaxis came to be known as *immediate hypersensitivity,* to distinguish its startling speed from the slower response of delayed-type hypersensitivity.

The swiftness of the anaphylactic response linked it to a third phenomenon. Charles Blackley had observed that his skin reactions to hay fever pollens took place very quickly, sometimes within minutes of exposure—suggesting that these reactions were also some form of immediate hypersensitivity. Anaphylaxis and allergic reactions were very different in both their symptoms and severity, but the apparent differences might well be only superficial. Researchers began to wonder if some immunologic link existed between these two immediate hypersensitivity reactions.

As early as 1906, immunologists suspected that allergic reactions might be caused by the interaction of allergens (antigens that trigger allergic responses) and certain substances circulating in the blood. And in 1921, two German physicians, Carl Prausnitz and Heinz Küstner, devised a way to test the hypothesis. They knew that if allergic responses were indeed the result of interactions between allergens and circulating substances, then it should be possible to transfer an allergy by injecting blood serum from an allergic individual into a nonallergic individual. As it happened, Küstner had a strong allergy to cooked fish, an allergy Prausnitz did not share. So a small amount of Küstner's serum was injected into Prausnitz's skin to sensitize him. The following day, the researchers injected an extract of cooked fish into the same site. Within a few minutes, the skin became swollen and reddened—exactly the allergic reaction

Blackley had observed when he scratched his skin with hay fever allergens. Injected with serum from Küstner, Prausnitz had become temporarily allergic to cooked fish.

The experiment proved that Küstner's sensitivity to fish had indeed been transmitted by a substance or substances circulating in the blood. Prausnitz remained sensitive to skin injections of fish extract for as long as two weeks after receiving injections of Küstner's serum. Then his sensitivity disappeared. The allergic response was closely limited to the site where the serum had been injected. Obviously, the circulating factor in Küstner's serum that transferred sensitivity to Prausnitz had fixed itself tightly to the tissues surrounding the injection site.

Within the next few years, researchers extended and clarified the findings of Küstner and Prausnitz. It was discovered that an allergic reaction to grass pollen could also be transferred through the serum of allergic individuals. Indeed, even anaphylactic responses could be induced in nonallergic animals by first injecting them with serum from a hypersensitive animal. And that finding at last established the link between the pioneer studies of Charles Blackley on hay fever and the studies of Richet and Portier on anaphylaxis. All *immediate hypersensitivity* reactions, including allergic responses and anaphylaxis, appeared to depend on one or more *circulating factors* in the blood of the allergic individual. These reactions were fundamentally different from the Koch phenomenon of *delayed-type hypersensitivity,* which was known to depend on the activation of *immune cells.*

But what was this circulating factor that caused allergic hypersensitivity? Years earlier, a number of researchers had guessed that circulating antibodies might be the cause of anaphylaxis and allergy. The unknown factor certainly seemed to have the specificity of an antibody. But in other ways it did not behave at all like one. It possessed none of the unique functional and chemical properties of known immunoglobulins. Immunoglobulins are stable at elevated temperatures, for example; the circulating factor was not. And unlike standard immunoglobulins, the factor remained firmly fixed to skin tissue for prolonged periods—up to several weeks, as Prausnitz and Küstner had discovered. With no real knowledge of what they were or how they functioned, investigators adopted the fuzzy term *reagins* to describe the antibody-like mediators of immediate hypersensitivity.

It was not until 1967 that the husband and wife team of Kimishige and Teruko Ishizaka finally isolated the mysterious factor. And as researchers had long suspected, reagins were antibodies—antibodies found in extremely small amounts in the blood, and possessing their own unique functional properties. Because the first group of reagins was purified from patients with an allergy to ragweed pollen, the Ishizakas named the new class of antibodies *immunoglobulin E,* after the allergen these antibodies recognized—ragweed allergen E.

Investigators were now sure that IgE, binding with an allergen, produced the varied symptoms of immediate hypersensitivity: localized skin reactions, difficulty in breathing, and even death from anaphylactic shock. But how did the binding of IgE and allergens have its effect? Two lines of research—one on a unique chemical compound and the other on a specialized group of cells—would finally converge, along with the discovery of IgE, to provide an answer.

At the turn of the century, with newly developed techniques for modifying the structure of molecules, chemists created a variety of new synthetic substances from naturally occurring molecules. Altering the common amino acid *histidine,* for example, they created a molecule called *beta-imidazolylethylamine,* more commonly known as *histamine.* In 1910, two British researchers, H. H. Dale and P. P. Laidlaw, became intrigued by a particular property of this synthetic molecule. Small amounts of histamine injected into rabbits would produce prostration, irregular breathing, and a weak or intermittent heartbeat. Histamine also brought about the rapid and profound contraction of smooth muscle tissue obtained from the lung—the same kind of muscle that contracts during an asthmatic attack. And higher concentrations of histamine could actually produce convulsive, obstructed breathing that sometimes caused the death of laboratory animals in a matter of seconds.

Dale and Laidlaw were struck by the similarity between the symptoms of histamine poisoning and those of anaphylaxis. But while they noted the striking similarities "as a point of interest and possible significance," they cautiously remarked that "the correspondence cannot be regarded as sufficient basis for theoretical speculation."*

Their phrasing was cautious, but their vision was prophetic.

For over the next forty years, evidence steadily accumulated to prove that the various symptoms of hay fever, asthma, and anaphylaxis were caused, in large part, by histamine. Investigators discovered that histamine could be isolated from fresh samples of liver, lung, and smooth muscle—proof that this potent substance, first observed as a synthetic molecule, actually occurred naturally in the body. And when small amounts

*Dale, H. H., and P. P. Laidlaw. 1910. The physiological action of imidazolyethylamine. *J. Physiol.* 41:318–344.

of histamine were injected directly under the skin, the site quickly became reddened and swollen—precisely the response Blackley had observed. Even more striking, investigators discovered that isolated smooth muscle undergoing the contractions associated with an allergic attack released histamine. Each time sensitized muscle was induced to contract by the addition of an allergen, histamine was soon observed in the broth surrounding the muscle. In the absence of the allergen, no histamine was found.

It now seemed clear that the binding of allergens and IgE antibodies stimulated the rapid release of histamine. The histamine itself was directly responsible for the symptoms of immediate hypersensitivity in allergic reactions. Only one piece of information was missing: the source of the histamine.

Between 1877 and 1879, a young doctoral student named Paul Ehrlich discovered the existence of two specialized populations of cells, one found in the connective tissue, the other in blood. Ehrlich called the connective tissue cells *mast cells,* and their counterparts in blood, *blood mast cells* (now referred to as *basophils*). These cells were remarkable in their structure: they contained large numbers of granules that stained red or violet when treated with a special dye. But even more remarkable was a curious property they possessed: in the presence of certain irritating substances, the stainable granules in these cells would disappear, and the cell itself would simply disintegrate. Some investigators began calling mast cells "explosive cells," because of their characteristic disintegration.

For more than half a century, mast cells remained nothing more than a scientific curiosity. No one could explain the nature or function of the stainable granules or the meaning of the strange explosion that took place when mast cells came in contact with certain irritants.

Then, in 1937, a group of researchers in Stockholm found a direct correlation between the numbers of mast cells found in tissue samples and the quantity of a large carbohydrate called *heparin* (known to inhibit the coagulation of blood) present in the tissue. Indeed, the researchers soon discovered that the stainable granules of mast cells contained considerable amounts of heparin. And within four years, other investigators discovered that during anaphylactic shock the mast cells of laboratory dogs disintegrated and released their stores of heparin, which then caused the failure of blood to clot, a characteristic symptom of anaphylaxis.

Researchers assumed that they had finally discovered the role of mast cells in the body—the production of heparin, which prevented the clotting of blood within blood vessels. In fact the evidence seemed so strongly to favor this hypothesis that a number of researchers began to call mast cells "heparinocytes." But heparin was only one of many substances released by mast cells. It was soon discovered that the amounts of histamine found in different tissues also correlated directly with the numbers of mast cells in those tissues. And subsequent experiments demonstrated that mast cells indeed released histamine as they disintegrated. The "heparinocyte" was also a "histaminocyte."

Since then, immunologists have discovered that the granules in mast cells actually release more than a dozen biologically active substances as they disintegrate. Some of the substances attract various cell types to the sites of mast cell disintegration. Others cause an increase in the flow of fluid and cells from the blood into the surrounding tissue. Still others, like histamine, are able to induce the smooth muscle contraction associated with asthmatic attacks. And recent studies indicate that one group of substances, called *leukotrienes,* may actually have a more potent and long-lasting role in asthma than that of histamine.

Most evidence suggests that mast cells play a role in normal inflammatory responses. Only when IgE molecules on their surface bind with certain allergens do these cells become involved in destructive allergic responses. Researchers have found that mast cells and basophils have large numbers of IgE antibody molecules bound to their surfaces. (As many as 500,000 IgE molecules can gather on a single cell.) These IgE molecules lie dormant on the surface of mast cells until they come in contact with an allergen they recognize. The binding of IgE and allergen then sets off a chain reaction within the mast cells and basophils that leads to their disintegration and the release of histamine, leukotrienes, heparin, and other substances. These substances cause the varied symptoms of hay fever and other allergies, asthma, and anaphylaxis.

When an allergic individual inhales ragweed pollen, for example, an explosion of immunologic activity takes place. Within the first five minutes, ragweed pollen grains will release over 90 percent of their allergens. These molecules quickly bind with IgE antibodies on the surface of mast cells in the lining of the nose. The allergen-IgE complexes that form then trigger the release of histamine and other substances responsible for the itchy eyes, runny nose, and nasal congestion of hay fever.

Quickly, the allergic response begins to amplify. Allergens, like any foreign antigen, will activate T cells passing through the site of the allergic response. These activated T cells stimulate B cells to produce high levels of additional IgE antibodies. At the same time, they release chemotactic factors, which attract basophils from the blood into the lining of the nose. Arriving basophils immediately bind with the newly produced IgE. And when these cells then come in contact with the allergen, they release new stores of histamine, heparin, and other mediators, amplifying the initial allergic response.

A similar immune response takes place during allergic reactions to a variety of other substances. During allergic reactions to food, for example, food allergens are released into the gastrointestinal tract. There they swiftly react with IgE antibodies in the lining of the intestines. The binding of IgE and allergens then releases histamine and other mediators responsible for the gastrointestinal symptoms of food allergies. Since food allergens can also be absorbed into the bloodstream, the binding of IgE and allergens may occur at sites far removed from the stomach or intestines—producing allergic responses that take the form of nasal congestion, difficulty in breathing, or skin rashes. In children, the great majority of food allergies are associated with five common food groups: milk, nuts, eggs, soybean, and wheat. In adults, fish are a major source of allergens that trigger allergic reactions.

Anaphylactic shock simply represents an exaggerated, and sometimes fatal, form of these same immunologic mechanisms. In Richet and Portier's early experiments with sea anemone toxins, for example, the first injection sensitized the laboratory dogs, producing IgE antibodies specific for the toxin. These antibodies became fixed to basophils and mast cells. The allergens injected during the second exposure then bound to the IgE molecules on these cells, causing a massive allergic response. The immunologic events underlying anaphylaxis are well known, but the question of why the same allergen will produce anaphylactic shock in one individual and only a mild allergic response in another still challenges immunologists.

Allergic reactions also appear to play a role in certain forms of asthma—although the precise relationship of allergy and asthma is still being explored. Almost a century ago, Charles Blackley recognized that his own allergic reactions to pollen sometimes escalated into the symptoms of asthma: wheezing, coughing, and constriction of the breathing passages. And about half of all people who suffer from asthma have allergies to one or more of the environmental allergens, including dust, animal dander, and pollens. Individuals with asthma generally have higher than normal levels of IgE, which may make them more prone to allergic reactions in general.

But asthma can also be triggered by a variety of nonimmunologic factors, like cold air, tobacco smoke, heightened emotion, and even exercise or excessive laughing. The one common feature of all asthmatic reactions is the unusual hypersensitivity of the smooth muscle of the breathing passages. Some researchers believe that repeated exposure to low levels of allergens may in fact be the cause of this heightened bronchial sensitivity.

Not all hay fever sufferers develop asthma, even after repeated exposure to hay fever allergens. And the reasons for the peculiar sensitivity of individuals with asthma may lie in the delicate relationship between the immune system and the nervous system, a relationship researchers are only now beginning to explore.

There is some evidence that asthmatics may lack normal nervous system control over bronchial muscle contraction and relaxation. In individuals with asthma, the nerve signals for contraction appear to dominate, keeping the bronchial muscle in a constant state of partial contraction. It may well be that this state of permanent partial contraction, coupled with a heightened sensitivity to allergens that in themselves can cause bronchial hypersensitivity, produces the conditions for asthma. Tentative findings have even suggested that nonimmunologic factors like cold air and exercise can cause mast cells and basophils to disintegrate, releasing their packets of histamine and other mediators. In an individual with asthma, the convergence of these factors may create a vicious circle in which both allergens and nonimmunologic stimuli irritate the already partially contracted bronchial muscles.

The discovery of IgE answered many questions about the immunologic events of an allergic response, but one fundamental mystery remained. Everyone has circulating IgE antibodies, yet only 10 percent of the population of the United States suffers from hay fever. For some people, a few grains of pollen can trigger a life-threatening asthmatic attack, while others could sleep on a bed of ragweed and experience no reaction at all. Why are some people allergic to certain substances, and others not?

Nearly half of all people with hay fever have at least one parent with some form of allergy or asthma. And children of parents who both have hay fever are far more likely to develop the allergy than children with only one allergic parent. But the job of *proving* these hereditary links has been very difficult, in part because of the number of uncontrollable variables. The specific form of allergy inherited by children, for example, may be very different from the allergies of their parents. And the lack of a standard method for measuring allergic sensitivity and the degree of prior exposure to an allergen have made it difficult for researchers to compare their findings. Most immunologists still believe, however, that a predisposition to allergy or asthma is inherited, passed along in the form of specific immune response genes that control the body's reaction to allergens in the environment.

Immune response genes contain information for producing specific proteins that determine how T and B cells will recognize and respond to foreign antigens. In the case of someone sensitive to ragweed pollen, for example, a specific form of immune response gene may provide information that allows B cells to produce IgE antibodies against ragweed allergen, which then bind to the surface of mast cells and basophils. And when ragweed pollen is encountered, antibody and allergen bind, triggering the cells to release histamine and other mediators. Most people have a slightly different form of this immune response gene—one that contains information for the production of suppressor T cells that can block the generation of IgE antibodies against ragweed pollen—so they have no allergic reaction at all.

Recently, research teams working in the United States and Japan have found that T cells produce two lymphokines which specifically control the production of IgE antibodies. One of these lymphokines, called *enhancing factor of allergy* or *IgE potentiating factor,* stimulates the body to produce IgE antibodies against specific allergens. A second lymphokine, called *suppressive factor of allergy* or *IgE-suppressive factor,* slows down or stops the production of IgE. The delicate balance of these two lymphokines may well dictate the level of IgE in the body —and the strength of an allergic response to allergens.

Whether a T cell will respond to a particular antigen by producing enhancing factor or suppressive factor is determined by the specific form of an immune response gene.

Probably the oldest treatment for allergy is simply one of avoidance: maintaining a respectable distance from the source of troubling allergens. That prescription is relatively easy to follow in the case of allergies to food or animal dander. But if the allergy is caused by pollen, dust, or other environmental allergens, it may be extremely difficult to avoid contact. In many cases, these allergy sufferers turn to desensitization therapy.

The technique of desensitization was first established in 1911, when two American researchers found that hay fever symptoms could be significantly reduced by injecting patients with steadily increasing amounts of a pollen extract. The researchers had no idea why the technique worked. Even today, after many years of experience with desensitization therapy, immunologists do not really understand the underlying immunologic activity. Allergens injected in small doses over a period of time induce the production of immunoglobulin G (IgG) antibodies. IgG antibodies may then bind with the allergens, blocking IgE molecules fixed to mast cells and basophils from binding with these allergens and forming the complexes that cause the release of histamine. Desensitization therapy may also serve to block T cells from recruiting basophils. If fewer basophils migrate to the site of an allergic reaction, then the levels of the mediators, and the symptoms they produce, would be correspondingly decreased.

Desensitization has proved successful against hay fever, allergies to insect bites, and other venom allergies. The therapeutic technique lessens the severity of symptoms in as many as 80 percent of the treated patients. But only a third of those experience permanent relief. In the rest, allergies recur, usually within a year to five years after the original treatment. And allergen injections must be used carefully. In rare instances, desensitization therapy can trigger anaphylactic shock. For allergic reactions like asthma, the risks of desensitization therapy seem to outweigh its potential benefits.

Drug therapy remains the most common treatment for allergies and asthma. Antihistamines, which block the effects of histamine on blood vessels and smooth muscle, are administered for the relief of hay fever and other environmental allergies. (Antihistamines are also used routinely to block the effects of histamine released during the inflammation that accompanies a common cold.) For asthmatic patients, the specific goal of drug therapy is to relax the bronchial smooth muscles so that breathing is not impaired. Normally, the nerves in the bronchial passage release a substance called *epinephrine,* which acts directly to relax the bronchial smooth muscles. *Beta-agonists* or *beta-adrenergic* drugs like metaproterenol sulfate (Alupent) or terbutaline (Brethine) mimic the action of epinephrine. A second class of drugs, called xanthines, are administered if asthma attacks occur regularly. And in some cases, physicians may administer *cromolyn sodium,* a drug which appears to block the release of histamine and other mediators. More severe asthmatic attacks may require the use of corticosteroids, drugs which reduce inflammation by directly suppressing the immune system.

Desensitization and drug therapies treat the symptoms of allergy and asthma. But as any allergy sufferer knows, they are by no means cures for the disease. Antihistamines, by blocking the effects of histamine, offer only partial relief. Mast cells and basophils release as many as ten active substances, including potent leukotrienes; and we have as yet no drugs which can block the specific action of many of these other mediators. While antihistamines are relatively weak drugs useful only in mild forms of hay fever, steroids are extremely potent; by blocking the specific function of certain immune cells, they suppress the full range of immune responses. Ideally, the most effective treatment against allergic reactions would specifically target their source—the immune response that regulates the synthesis of IgE.

With the discovery of the two lymphokines involved in the stimulation and suppression of IgE production—IgE potentiating factor and IgE suppressive factor—investigators have identified two of the important controls that regulate allergic responses. And research is already underway to purify and produce sufficient quantities of these potent molecules for further study and testing. Before long, immunologists may learn how to administer IgE suppressive factor in order to turn off an allergic response. They may even decipher the lymphokine commands that stimulate the production of IgE suppressive factor, which may enable physicians to stop allergic immune responses even before they begin, by using the language of the immune system itself.

eleven

IN SELF-DEFENSE

We no longer find ourselves lost on a boundless sea . . . we have already caught a distinct glimpse of the land which we hope, nay, which we expect, will yield rich treasures for biology and therapeutics.

PAUL EHRLICH, 1900

With Metchnikoff's discovery of specialized cells that could attack and destroy invading pathogens, scientists had their first glimpse into the power and scope of the system that defends the body against disease. And as immunologists have gradually sharpened the focus of their research down to the smallest details of that system—antigens and antigen receptors, lymphokines, and even the genes that program our susceptibility to disease—they have come away with a constantly renewed sense of wonder at the intricate mechanisms of the human immune system.

Our power to see more closely and more clearly has often come from important technological advances. Leeuwenhoek's handmade light microscope gave him, for the first time, the power to see the "little animalcules" called bacteria, protozoa, and fungi. The invention of the electron microscope and the development of cell culture techniques enabled researchers to see the structure and activity of viruses. Recombinant DNA techniques have extended our powers in many profound ways —offering, among other breakthroughs, a way to produce large quantities of lymphokines for analysis and clinical testing.

And in recent years, immunologists have gained another significant research tool—one that has enabled them to dissect the innermost components of the immune system with unprecedented precision. The development of this new technology began, curiously, with a particular form of cancer. Researchers had long been aware that B cells, like any other cells in the body, can become cancerous. In the 1960s, researchers discovered techniques to isolate B cell tumors from laboratory animals and adapt them to grow in culture dishes. As long as these tumors, called *myelomas,* were supplied with nutrients, they would grow indefinitely—like all tumor cells. Myelomas were of special interest to researchers, however, because these "immortalized" cells continued to produce antibodies. Each myeloma, like its normal B cell counterpart, will produce a homogeneous population of antibodies. Proliferating indefinitely in a nutrient broth, they provided researchers for the first time with a large source of antibodies for the study of antibody structure and function.

There was just one problem. Investigators had no way to know which specific antigen a myeloma-produced antibody recognized. A myeloma is derived from a single random B cell, and there are an estimated one million B cell subpopulations, each producing antibodies specific to a unique antigen. To determine which antigen a particular myeloma-produced antibody recognized, researchers would have to test hundreds of thousands of possible antigens. The chances of success would be one in a million—and this monumental task would have to be repeated with each and every myeloma-produced antibody. For researchers interested in studying the physical interaction of *specific* antibodies and antigens, myelomas were of little value.

Then, in the early 1970s, George Köhler and Cesar Milstein, working in Cambridge, England, found a solution—a way to create myelomas that would produce specific, identifiable antibodies. They took advantage of a new technology called *hybridization* or *cell fusion,* which enabled investigators to fuse two cells together to form a single cell exhibiting properties associated with both of the fusion partners. Their idea was to fuse a myeloma cell with a normal B cell that produced antibody specific for a known antigen. If the technique succeeded, they would create a hybrid cell which combined the ability of the myeloma to grow indefinitely with the ability of the normal B cell to produce an antibody against a known antigen.

Köhler and Milstein began their experiment by immunizing laboratory mice with red blood cells taken from sheep—cells which are strongly antigenic in mice. The procedure generated large populations of B cells producing antibodies which targeted antigens on the sheep red blood cells. The B cells were then removed from the mice and fused with myelomas. When the researchers began to test the new hybrid cells, they were excited to find that several of them were indeed producing antibodies against antigens on the red blood cells of sheep. And because one of the fusion partners was a myeloma, these hybrid cells were able to grow indefinitely, producing large quantities of a single antibody specific to a known antigen.

Before long, researchers discovered that they could fuse a normal B cell with a myeloma that had lost its ability to produce antibody—insuring that the antibody produced by the hybrid would always be that of the normal B cell fusion partner. The products of this revolutionary technique—homogeneous antibodies produced by a single population or *clone* of cells, each one identical to the others—were called *monoclonal antibodies.* And with the development of these tailor-made antibodies, a completely new field of immunologic research was born.

Although the effects of an immune response, like the skin reaction to tuberculin, may be visible to the naked eye, the cellular and molecular components at work in the immune system are extremely minute. While scientists have long been able to see macrophages under the microscope, for example, they could not see or easily isolate a lymphokine such as interleukin 1. While they could watch the rapid destruction of a foreign skin graft, immunologists had no way to see or easily characterize the histocompatibility antigens that initiated the rejection process itself.

With the development of monoclonal antibodies, however, investigators suddenly had the power to isolate and study many of these smallest components of the immune system in precise detail.

In the early years of lymphokine research, for example, the purification of a specific lymphokine required as many as twelve separate steps, and with each step a little more of the precious substance was lost. Using monoclonal antibodies, however, researchers have successfully purified lymphokines like interleukin 2 and gamma interferon in a single step. Monoclonal antibodies can be created that will recognize any specific protein molecule. And what makes antibodies particularly useful is their ability to bind to the protein molecule they recognize. Researchers have developed monoclonal antibodies that recognize and bind to a specific lymphokine protein molecule. These antibodies are then attached to beads of inert material, several thousand molecules to a single bead. The beads are placed in glass columns. When the broth from a culture of immune cells (broth containing a number of lymphokines secreted by the cells) is poured through the columns, the monoclonal antibodies bind the specific lymphokine molecules they recognize. And because the antibodies are held in place by the inert beads, they separate the targeted lymphokine molecules and hold them within the column while the other factors pass through. Using certain chemical techniques, researchers can then release the bound lymphokines and collect them.

In some experiments, researchers use this technique to isolate and study a particular lymphokine molecule; in others, researchers have removed a single lymphokine from a culture broth in order to study how its absence affects particular immune responses.

In the first excitement of his new discovery, Leeuwenhoek observed that "there are more animals living in the scum on the teeth of a man's mouth, than there are men in the whole kingdom."* With the help of monoclonal antibodies, immunologists have been equally excited by the discovery of new

*Quoted in Stanier, R. Y., M. Doudoroff, and E. A. Adelberg. 1963. *The Microbial World.* Englewood Cliffs, N.J.: Prentice-Hall.

and important regulatory substances, as well as immune cell subpopulations never before observed. Previously unknown subpopulations of B cells have been identified by the production of monoclonal antibodies that bind unique molecules on the surface of these cells, trapping them and separating them for study.

Indeed, like a miniature laser in the hand of a brain surgeon, monoclonal antibodies are a tool that enables immunologists to isolate the smallest components of immune response with exquisite accuracy. Using this new technology, researchers have already begun to unlock one of the great remaining mysteries of the immune system: the chemical nature of the T cell receptor, the surface molecule that enables a T cell to recognize a specific antigen. With more than one million different T cell subpopulations, each programmed to recognize a single antigen, it has been virtually impossible for researchers to identify unique antigen receptors. With the use of monoclonal antibodies, however, researchers can now isolate a T cell receptor specific for a known antigen in order to study its unique chemical makeup.

The potential of monoclonal antibodies in clinical medicine may prove to be as far-reaching as the potential of lymphokine therapy. In laboratory studies, for example, researchers have cured mice of a virus-induced leukemia (cancer of the white blood cells) by inoculating them with small amounts of a monoclonal antibody that specifically targets a viral antigen. The antibodies seek out and bind to the cancer cells, initiating the full range of antibody and cell-mediated responses against them—but without causing harm to the normal cells of the body. By developing monoclonal antibodies that recognize antigens unique to human tumor cells, researchers hope to use the same technique for treating cancer patients. In fact, antibodies have already been developed that recognize unique lung tumor antigens, as well as antigens of certain human leukemia cells.

Monoclonal antibodies may also provide a useful technique for the early diagnosis of cancer. Tumor cells are known to shed cell surface antigens, which eventually make their way into the bloodstream. The level of these specific antigens in the blood relates, in a general way, to the number of tumor cells in the body. Monoclonal antibodies have enabled researchers to isolate these specific tumor antigens and measure their concentration in blood, providing a new way to determine the relative number of cancer cells in the body. In a recent study, investigators developed a monoclonal antibody that targets an antigen found on a specific human gastrointestinal tumor. Adding this antibody to blood samples taken from thirty-three patients with the cancer, researchers were able to detect the shed antigens in more than two-thirds of the patients—confirming that this technique may be useful in detecting cancer in its early stages.

Perhaps the most exciting clinical potential for monoclonal antibodies lies in the use of *immunotoxins.* By attaching specific toxic substances to monoclonal antibodies, immunologists have created a kind of biologic bomb with an extremely accurate guidance system. When a monoclonal antibody carrying a toxic antitumor drug selectively binds to a tumor cell, the drug enters the cell and swiftly destroys it without affecting healthy cells in the body. Immunotoxins have already been used with considerable success in laboratory studies on animals with leukemia, melanoma, and a number of other forms of cancer.

Researchers hope that immunotoxins may also be of value

in preventing graft versus host disease following bone marrow transplants. In a recent study, investigators developed an immunotoxin that targets an antigen found on the mature T cells of laboratory mice—the principal cells involved in graft versus host disease. Added to cultures of bone marrow cells, the immunotoxin eliminated these populations of mature T cells. Researchers then transplanted the cleansed bone marrow into mice with histocompatibility antigens unrelated to the donors. The results were impressive. While the injection of untreated bone marrow uniformly resulted in serious graft versus host disease in the genetically unrelated mice, the injection of treated bone marrow was accepted by the mice without a single instance of graft versus host disease. In the future, researchers may use this approach routinely in human bone marrow transplant patients.

Immunotoxins may eventually be used to avert the rejection of transplanted organs and tissues as well. Rejection is carried out by specific populations of T cells—those that bear receptors which recognize certain foreign histocompatibility antigens. It may be possible to develop immunotoxins that target only these receptors on the transplant recipient's T cells. With precise accuracy, immunotoxins would destroy only the T cells involved in rejection, leaving the full range of other T cells to continue the defense against microbial pathogens.

In the same way, immunotoxins that target specific T cell receptors may one day play a role in the treatment of allergies and asthma. Immunotoxins directed against T cells that recognize ragweed pollen, for example, would be able to destroy those T cells responsible for initiating the production of IgE against the pollen. Without the presence of these IgE antibodies, mast cells and basophils would not be stimulated to release their stores of histamine, leukotrienes, and the other mediators of allergy and asthma.

We stand at the edge of a new frontier in immunology and medicine. Monoclonal antibodies, with their ability to target specific cells and substances with perfect precision, and lymphokines, with their power to control and alter the course of an immune response, represent two of the most important directions that future research will take. But a biologic system as complex as the immune system can be studied and understood from many different perspectives. As some researchers explore the therapeutic potential of lymphokines and monoclonal antibodies, others are expanding the frontiers of immunologic research in new directions—studying the immune system not only in its parts, but in its relationship to other systems of the body, and to the body as a whole.

The immune system exists in a delicate balance with other regulatory systems in the body. The fever control center of the central nervous system, for example, is regulated and controlled, at least in part, by the release of interleukin 1 during an immune response against pathogens. The constriction of bronchial smooth muscle in individuals with asthma is dictated by a complex interplay of signals from both the immune and nervous systems. The balance of male and female hormones, controlled by the endocrine system, appears to have a significant influence on the activity of immune cells in autoimmune disorders.

And there may be more profound and subtle links between the immune system and the nervous and endocrine systems. Researchers have known for some time, for example, that high levels of stress can significantly increase the incidence of cancer and serious infectious illnesses in laboratory animals. And latent human viruses like herpes simplex appear to be triggered, in some way, by periods of stress. The severity and frequency of allergic and asthmatic responses are also powerfully influenced by stress or strong emotional reactions. Stress can even affect the ability of the immune system to respond to a graft of foreign tissue. In one recent study, for example, investigators found that mice subjected to high levels of stress exhibited very weak graft rejection responses—evidence of a general suppression of immune responsiveness.

The mechanisms which link the immune, endocrine, and nervous systems are not well understood. Some studies suggest that stress may depress the functioning of T cells; others point to weakened B cell responses; still others have indicated that the activity of natural killer cells and phagocytes may be impaired in animals exposed to high levels of stress. Researchers *have* discovered, however, that high levels of stress can cause the adrenal gland to release increased amounts of cortisol, a potent steroid. Cortisol has a number of profound effects on the body's metabolism. But what interests immunologists is its powerful ability to suppress immune and inflammatory responses. Cortisol-like steroids are administered routinely to transplant patients and patients with serious autoimmune diseases or asthma, specifically to suppress the immune system. Researchers do not know exactly how cortisol produces its effect, but recent studies have suggested that steroids may completely block the production of interleukin 1, inhibiting the subsequent cascade of lymphokines that control cell-mediated and antibody responses. The release of cortisol by the adrenal gland, an endocrine organ, is ultimately controlled by the brain.

Other endocrine hormones may also be involved in the development and functioning of the immune system. Insulin, growth hormone, and thyroid hormone have all been shown to affect the activities of specific immune cells. And there is intriguing evidence that certain chemicals produced by the brain itself may have a powerful effect on immune responses. Two classes of chemicals, called *endorphins* and *enkephalins,* are known to influence our perception of pain. Released by the brain, both of these naturally occurring pain killers function very much like the narcotic morphine. But endorphins and enkephalins have another potent effect: they enhance both the activation of T cells and the ability of natural killer cells to destroy tumors. Investigators have discovered that moderate exercise stimulates the production of endorphins and enkephalins, suggesting an immunologic link between exercise and good health.

Research into the interactions of the nervous, endocrine, and immune systems is still in its infancy. The little we already know has given researchers a breathtaking sense of the wonder of the human body at work. The communications network between the three systems may be as complex as lymphokine communications within the immune system itself. Future research into this network will no doubt yield important new insights into how distinct biologic systems within the body work together.

From the smallest antigen capable of triggering an immune response to the complex interplay between lymphocytes and the nervous system, the body's mechanisms of self-defense are steadily yielding their intimate secrets. In the last decade alone, exciting research breakthroughs have greatly expanded our understanding of human immune responses. But the basic discoveries of immunology have not come easily. Years, and sometimes decades, have passed between a chance observation and the full understanding of its nature and implications.

When Elie Metchnikoff poked a rose thorn into a starfish larva, he had no idea of the many roles that phagocytes would ultimately be found to play in the defense of the human body. Biologists at the turn of the century certainly could not have predicted that their frustrating attempts to grow tumors in mice would one day lead to the discovery of histocompatibility antigens and the enhanced survival of heart and kidney transplants. And the puzzle of allergy and asthma was probably far from the minds of the chemists who transformed histidine, a common amino acid, into a new and unique substance called histamine.

There is a fundamental paradox in scientific research. Scientists carefully plan their experiments to prevent any unforeseen complications that might impair the interpretation of experimental findings. Yet it is the unforeseen and often surprising experimental result that creates sudden insight and new understanding. Confident of their methods and approach when they injected laboratory dogs with sea anemone toxin in the hope of immunizing them, Richet and Portier were truly shocked by the violent deaths of several of the animals. But their surprise quickly gave way to insight: they had uncovered a new immunologic phenomenon, anaphylaxis. Robert Koch was just as surprised to see the reddening and swelling of the skin that followed a second exposure to tuberculin. He could not explain the reasons for the distinct reaction—but the mystery of the Koch phenomenon would ultimately lead other investigators to the discovery of lymphokines. And before long, lymphokine therapy may offer substantial hope for patients with a wide range of diseases, from allergies and asthma to Acquired Immune Deficiency Syndrome.

No one can chart in advance the exact course that will lead from a breakthrough in basic research to its application in a practical, life-saving therapy. No one can place a precise value on an isolated finding, an individual insight, a small breakthrough in understanding. The chance observation noted and dismissed by one scientist may be seized upon by another as the decisive clue that solves some central mystery. The work of the many great scientists in immunology—Elie Metchnikoff, Louis Pasteur, Robert Koch, Karl Landsteiner, Paul Ehrlich, Sir Peter Medawar, and many others—has borne this out. In the end, each new experiment, each new finding, each step forward in immunologic research advances not only our basic understanding of the wonder and complexity of the human immune system, but also, in the truest sense, our own self-defense.

GLOSSARY

ABO blood group antigens Major protein antigens present on the surface of red blood cells. There are four ABO blood types: A, B, AB, and O.

Acquired Immune Deficiency Syndrome (AIDS) An extremely serious immunodeficiency disease caused by a viral pathogen. The disease is characterized by a large number of opportunistic infections and Kaposi's sarcoma.

allergen A substance that stimulates IgE synthesis or interacts with IgE to produce an immediate hypersensitivity reaction and the symptoms of allergy or asthma.

anaphylaxis A severe, life-threatening allergic reaction caused by the release of histamine and other substances from mast cells and basophils.

antibody A protein produced by B cells that specifically recognizes and binds to a single antigen and is involved in the neutralization or destruction of that antigen.

antigen A substance that is recognized as foreign by immune cells or antibodies and can stimulate an immune response.

autoantibody An antibody directed against other antibodies in the body or against self-antigens on host cells.

autoimmunity A state of abnormal immune reactivity against self-antigens.

basophil A circulating cell that releases histamine and other mediators in response to irritants or the binding of IgE-allergen complexes on its surface.

B cell A cell that produces an antibody against a specific antigen.

cellular immunity A form of immunity that involves cells—phagocytes, T cells, and natural killer cells.

chemotactic factor A lymphokine released by immune cells that recruits specific populations of immune and nonimmune cells to sites of immune or inflammatory responses.

complement A group of approximately fifteen proteins found in blood that interact with antibodies to produce holes in foreign cells or virus-infected or cancerous host cells.

cyclosporin A A potent and specific immunosuppressive drug currently being used in transplant surgery.

delayed-type hypersensitivity A slowly developing immune response (easily observed on the skin) mediated by immune cells—phagocytes and T cells—but not antibodies.

encephalomyelitis An inflammation of the brain and spinal cord.

endotoxin A cell wall component shed from some bacteria that can indirectly produce widespread tissue damage by generating an exaggerated and potentially lethal response from immune cells.

enhancing antibodies Antibodies produced in response to the presence of a foreign tissue—a fetus, tumor cells, or sperm, for example—that protect such tissue from immunologic destruction.

exotoxin A substance released by pathogenic bacteria that can directly damage specific cells or tissues in the body.

granulocyte A cell (also termed a neutrophil) that is primarily involved in the engulfment of pathogenic microorganisms, inert particles like asbestos, and cellular debris.

helper T cell A T cell that stimulates T cell growth, B cell antibody production and macrophage activation via the release of specific lymphokine signals.

histocompatibility antigens Cell surface proteins on immune cells that are specifically involved in the recognition of foreign antigens by T cells, but which themselves can serve as very potent stimuli for graft rejection.

histamine A small protein molecule released by mast cells and basophils that is responsible for many of the symptoms of allergic responses.

human leukocyte antigens (HLA) Human histocompatibility proteins present on the surface of immune cells that control graft rejection, susceptibility to various diseases, and the recognition of specific antigens.

humoral immunity A form of immunologic defense that involves the action of antibodies and complement.

IgE potentiating factor A lymphokine (also termed enhancing factor of allergy) that selectively stimulates the production of IgE antibodies by B cells.

IgE suppressive factor A lymphokine (also termed suppressive factor of allergy) that selectively inhibits the production of IgE antibodies by B cells.

immediate hypersensitivity A very rapid allergic response mediated by IgE antibodies. The binding of allergen-IgE complexes to mast cells and basophils triggers the release of histamine and other mediators of allergy and asthma.

immune response genes A select group of histocompatibility genes that determine the nature of the response to specific antigens. These genes may also regulate the susceptibility of an individual to infectious, autoimmune, and allergic diseases.

immune tolerance A state of nonresponsiveness to a specific antigen.

immunoglobulin Another term used to describe an antibody. There are five classes of immunoglobulins: IgG, IgM, IgD, IgA, and IgE.

immunotoxin A specific monoclonal antibody attached to a toxic drug.

impedin A substance (also termed aggressin) released by pathogenic bacteria that interferes with the activities of immune cells and antibodies.

inflammation The body's normally protective repair response to tissue damage. An inflammatory response may be nonspecific or antigen-specific, depending on the nature of the agent responsible for the tissue damage—for example, a knife wound versus the injection of tuberculin under the skin.

interferons A family of proteins produced by immune and nonimmune cells that not only protect cells from virus-mediated destruction, but also enhance the activities of macrophages, killer T cells, and natural killer cells.

interleukin 1 A lymphokine produced by macrophages that activates T cells as well as a variety of nonimmune cells involved in inflammatory responses.

interleukin 2 A lymphokine produced by T cells that stimulates the growth of T cells and natural killer cells.

killer T cell A T cell that specifically targets and destroys virus-infected cells and cancer cells.

leukotrienes Small molecules released by mast cells and basophils that may be responsible for a considerable portion of the bronchial smooth muscle constriction during asthmatic attacks.

lymph node An organ of the immune system in which T cells and B cells are activated by specific antigens.

lymphokines Proteins secreted by immune cells that function as a communication link between immune and nonimmune cells involved in immune and inflammatory responses. Some lymphokines may have a direct killing effect on cancer cells.

macrophage An immune cell that can engulf pathogenic micoorganisms and activate a large number of distinct cell types involved in immune responses. Interleukin 1 is an important lymphokine signal produced by macrophages.

mast cell A cell found in tissues that, like basophils, releases histamine and other substances upon stimulation by irritants or IgE-allergen complexes.

memory cell Long-lived T and B cells that specifically recognize and react against a specific antigen to which the immune system has been exposed.

migration inhibitory factor A lymphokine produced by T cells that inhibits the movement of macrophages.

monoclonal antibodies Homogeneous antibodies produced by a single population or clone of immortalized B cells that are created by the fusion of normal and tumor B cells.

myelin basic protein A component of myelin, the protective sheath that surrounds nerve cells in the central nervous system. Myelin basic protein is a major antigenic trigger in experimental encephalomyelitis and multiple sclerosis.

natural killer cells Non-T cells that do not require a prior state of activation in order to successfully attack and destroy virus-infected cells and cancer cells.

normal flora The population of microorganisms that reside on or in the human body and do not pose a health hazard in healthy immunocompetent individuals.

osteoclast activating factor A lymphokine that activates osteoclasts, cells that are involved in the routine maintenance of bone structure.

pathogen A disease-causing microorganism—a virus, bacterium, protozoan, mold or yeast, or helminth.

phagocyte A cell—either a macrophage or granulocyte—that engulfs pathogens or inert particles like silica or asbestos.

reagins A term used to describe IgE antibodies.

rheumatoid factors Autoantibodies produced against other circulating antibodies. Rheumatoid factors are commonly detected in rheumatoid arthritis and systemic lupus erythematosus.

spleen An organ of the immune system containing large numbers of T and B cells.

slow viruses Viruses that can exist within the tissues of the body for extremely long periods without inducing detectable symptoms.

suppressor T cell A T cell that inhibits the generation or progression of immune responses to specific antigens.

synovial cells Nonimmune cells in the joints of rheumatoid arthritic patients that release inflammatory substances that cause tissue destruction and pain.

T cell receptor A protein present on the surface of each T cell that specifically recognizes and binds a unique antigen. The binding of an antigen to a T cell receptor is an important trigger for the activation of that cell.

thymus An organ of the immune system in which T cell precursors from the bone marrow mature into active helper, killer, and suppressor T cells.

trophoblast The fetal-derived membrane separating fetal and maternal tissues.

tumor necrosis factor A lymphokine that is probably secreted by macrophages and which has been shown to cause the destruction of some solid tumors in laboratory animals.

vaccine Weakened (attenuated) or dead microorganisms used as an antigen to produce long-term immunity to the pathogenic form of a microorganism.

SELECTED SOURCES

AUGUST, J. T. (1982). *Monoclonal Antibodies in Drug Development.* American Society for Pharmacology and Experimental Therapeutics, Bethesda, MD.

BARRETT, J. T. (1983). *Textbook of Immunology. An Introduction to Immunochemistry and Immunobiology.* C. V. Mosby Company, St. Louis, Mo.

BEER, A. E., and R. E. BILLINGHAM. (1976). *The Immunobiology of Mammalian Reproduction.* Prentice-Hall, Englewood Cliffs, N.J.

CAHILL, K. M. (1983). *The AIDS Epidemic.* St. Martin's Press, New York.

CLARK, W. R. (1983). *The Experimental Foundations of Modern Immunology.* John Wiley & Sons, New York.

COHEN, S., E. PICK, and J. J. OPPENHEIM (eds.). (1979). *Biology of the Lymphokines.* Academic Press, New York.

DHINDSA, D. S., and G. F. B. SCHUMACHER (eds.). (1980). *Immunological Aspects of Infertility and Fertility Regulation.* Elsevier/-North-Holland, New York.

FERRONE, S., E. S. CURTONI, and S. GORINI (eds.). (1979). *HLA Antigens in Clinical Medicine and Biology.* Garland STPM Press, New York.

HOGARTH, P. J. (1982). *Immunological Aspects of Mammalian Reproduction.* Blackie & Sons, Ltd., Glasgow.

LACHMANN, P. J., and D. K. PETERS (eds.). (1982). *Clinical Aspects of Immunology.* Blackwell Scientific Publications, Oxford, England.

LICHTENSTEIN, L. M., and K. F. AUSTEN. (1977). *Asthma. Physiology, Immunopharmacology, and Treatment.* Academic Press, New York.

LICHTENSTEIN, L. M., and A. FAUCI (1983). *Current Therapy in Allergy and Immunology 1983–1984.* B. C. Decker, Inc., Philadelphia, PA.

OPPENHEIM, J. J., and S. COHEN (1983). *Interleukins, Lymphokines, and Cytokines. Proceedings of the Third International Lymphokine Workshop.* Academic Press, New York.

PAUL, W. E., C. G. FATHMAN, and H. METZGER (eds.). (1983). *Annual Review of Immunology* (v. 1), Annual Reviews, Inc., Palo Alto, CA.

SAMTER, M. (ed.). (1978) *Immunological Diseases.* Little, Brown & Company, Boston.

STANIER, R. Y., M. DOUDOROFF, E. A. ADELBERG (1963). *The Microbial World.* Prentice-Hall, Englewood Cliffs, N.J.

STANWORTH, D. R. (1973). *Immediate Hypersensitivity. The Molecular Basis of the Allergic Response.* Elsevier/North-Holland, New York.

STITES, D. P., J. D. STOBO, H. H. FUDENBERG, J. V. WELLS (eds.). (1982). *Basic & Clinical Immunology.* Lange Medical Publications, Los Altos, CA.

VOLK, W. A. (1982). *Essentials of Medical Microbiology.* J. P. Lippincott Company, Philadelphia, PA.

DE WECK, A. L., F. KRISTENSEN, and M. LANDY (eds.). (1980). *Biochemical Characterization of Lymphokines. Proceedings of the Second International Lymphokine Workshop.* Academic Press, New York.

WHITE, D. J. G. (ed.). (1982). *Cyclosporin A.* Elsevier Biomedical Press, Amsterdam.

ZIFF, M., G. P. VELO, and S. GORINI. (eds.). (1982). "Rheumatoid Arthritis." In: *Advances in Inflammation Research* (v. 3), Raven Press, New York.

Recent research articles in the following scientific journals were also used as source material:

Acta Medica Scandinavica
American Journal of Clinical Oncology
American Journal of Medical Science
Annals of Surgery
Arthritis and Rheumatism
British Medical Journal
Cancer Research
Cancer Treatment Reviews
Cellular Immunology
Clinical and Experimental Immunology
Clinical Immunology and Immunopathology
Clinical Oncology
Immunological Reviews
International Journal of Cancer
Journal of the American Medical Association
Journal of the National Cancer Institute
Lymphokines
Nature
Proceedings of the National Academy of Sciences (USA)
Proceedings of the Royal Society of London
Science
The European Journal of Immunology
The Journal of Experimental Medicine
The Journal of Immunology
The Lancet
The New England Journal of Medicine
Transplantation Proceedings

INDEX

a

q

r

s

t